O9-AID-401

STRONG WOMEN

STAY SLIM

By the same authors

STRONG WOMEN STAY YOUNG

Miriam E. Nelson, Ph.D.

with Sarah Wernick, Ph.D.

Strong Women

Stay Slim

MENUS AND RECIPES
BY STEVEN RAICHLEN
ILLUSTRATIONS BY WENDY WRAY

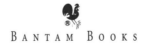

BANTAM BOOKS

NEW YORK TORONTO
LONDON SYDNEY AUCKLAND

STRONG WOMEN STAY SLIM
A Bantam Book / April 1998
All rights reserved.
Copyright © 1998 by Miriam E. Nelson, Ph.D., and Sarah Wernick, Ph.D.
Section IV, Menus and Recipes, copyright 1998 by Steven Raichlen
Illustrations by Wendy Wray/Vicki Morgan Associates, NYC

The PAR-Q test on page 98, from the 1994 revised version of the Physical Activity
Readiness Questionnaire (PAR-Q & YOU), has been reprinted with permission from the
Canadian Society for Exercise Physiology, Inc. The PAR-Q & YOU is a copyrighted,
pre-exercise screen owned by the Canadian Society for Exercise Physiology.

The Body Mass Index table on page 91 has been adapted with permission from
George A. Bray, M.D., copyright © 1988.

The statements in the box on page 94 have been adapted with permission from
Anorexia Nervosa and Related Eating Disorders, Inc.

The research described in this book has been funded at least in part with federal funds
from the U.S. Department of Agriculture, Agricultural Research Service. The contents of
this publication do not necessarily reflect the views or policies of the U.S. Department of
Agriculture, nor does mention of trade names, commercial products, or organizations
imply endorsement by the U.S. Government.

No part of this book may be reproduced or transmitted in any form or by any means,
electronic or mechanical, including photocopying, recording, or by any information
storage and retrieval system, without permission in writing from the publisher. For
information address: Bantam Books.

Library of Congress Cataloging-in-Publication Data

Nelson, Miriam E.
Strong women stay slim / Miriam E. Nelson, with Sarah Wernick.
p.   cm.
Includes index.
ISBN 0-553-10931-6
1. Reducing exercises.   2. Weight training for women.   3. Reducing diets—Recipes.
4. Exercise for women.   5. Physical fitness for women.   I. Wernick, Sarah.   II. Title.
RA781.6.N45   1998
613.7'1'082—dc21   97-44179
CIP

Published simultaneously in the United States and Canada

Bantam Books are published by Bantam Books, a division of Bantam Doubleday Dell
Publishing Group, Inc. Its trademark, consisting of the words "Bantam Books" and the
portrayal of a rooster, is Registered in U.S. Patent and Trademark Office and in other
countries. Marca Registrada. Bantam Books, 1540 Broadway, New York, New York 10036.

PRINTED IN THE UNITED STATES OF AMERICA

BVG 10 9 8 7 6 5 4 3 2 1

CONTENTS

▼   ▼   ▼   ▼

For my past and present students

▼ ▼ ▼ ▼

ACKNOWLEDGMENTS

▼ ▼ ▼ ▼

This book would not have been possible without the expertise and assistance of many people. I want to thank these individuals for their generous support.

During the research and writing of this book, I was fortunate to have the help of two superb assistants:

Jennifer Layne, M.S., C.S.C.S., my extraordinary research associate, was part of this project from conception to completion. Jennifer helped me identify women to test the program and discuss their experiences. She worked with me in developing the exercises, and she led the exercise segments of our focus group meetings. I benefited tremendously from her knowledge, experience, and creativity—as well as from her encouragement and support.

Melissa Allen, M.S., R.D., my very talented graduate student and research dietitian, worked with me on the nutrition program. She was invaluable in the design of the food plan, and she led the nutrition segments of the focus group, working closely with participants. Melissa also located women to test the program and share their stories. Her expertise, ingenuity, and hard work were greatly appreciated.

I've had enormous help from my colleagues at Tufts University: Ronenn Roubenoff, M.D., Irwin Rosenberg, M.D., Susan Roberts, Sc.D., Jacob Selhub, Ph.D., Jose Ordovas, Ph.D., Jeffrey Blumberg, Ph.D., Carmen Castaneda Sceppa, M.D., Ph.D., Christina Economos, Ph.D., Roger Fielding, Ph.D., Charles Pu, M.D., and Jeanne Goldberg, Ph.D., R.D. These leading scientists shared their expertise and their time, brainstorming the concepts of this program, updating me on their research, and reviewing chapters of the manuscript as they were written. I've also benefited from the kind assistance of colleagues outside Tufts. Steven Blair, P.E.D., of the Cooper Institute for Aerobics Research in Dallas, Texas, answered my many detailed questions regarding physical activity and health. Eric Poehlman, Ph.D., of the University of Vermont, provided valuable information about the determinants of energy metabolism.

Julia Robarts, R.D., did a painstaking review of the menus and recipes, to make sure the nutrition information was accurate. I also want to acknowledge the expert assistance of my past research technician, Sharon Bortz, M.S., R.D., who helped to design and lead the pilot research project that inspired this program. And I'm very grateful to Mike Pimentel, L.A.T.C., C.S.C.S., for his extensive efforts coordinating the photo shoot for the illustrations.

A special thanks to Larry Lindner and the *Tufts University Health & Nutrition Letter* for continuing to bring our research findings to the general public.

For their support, I also want to thank the Brookdale Foundation and the Mary Ingraham Bunting Institute at Radcliffe College, where I am currently a Bunting Fellow.

I'm very grateful to the many people who helped me translate what I've learned in the laboratory into a practical book for women:

I am forever indebted to my collaborator and dear friend, Sarah Wernick, who worked with me day in and day out to get this book written. I am in awe of her talent. She was always able to push me further to develop interesting scientific facts and personal stories for our readers.

I want to thank Steven Raichlen, cookbook author extraordinaire, for his brilliant menus and recipes—proof that healthy can be delicious.

Wendy Wray has graced the pages of this book with her illustrations. I appreciate not only her artistry but also her careful attention to detail.

Toni Burbank, my editor at Bantam, and her associates have been incredibly supportive. Toni is a rare and wonderful editor who is able to find the magical balance between respecting the writer's vision and advocating for the readers' needs. I benefited tremendously from her many helpful suggestions. I also want to give heartfelt thanks to Robin Michaelson, Toni's very able assistant, for all the help she so competently and cheerfully provided.

My literary agent, Wendy Weil, has been an enthusiastic advocate for this book. I'm so grateful for her expertise and her encouragement.

Three talented writers critiqued the manuscript as it became a book. My gratitude to Sally Wendkos Olds, Barbara Sofer, and Anita Bartholemew for their valuable comments and suggestions. Special thanks to my colleague William Lockeretz, Ph.D., who carefully reviewed the entire manuscript for both technical and grammatical accuracy.

Working with women in the laboratory and in our focus groups has been one of the most enjoyable parts of my work. My gratitude to the dedicated volunteers who have so generously given their time to participate in my research. A warm thank-you to the wonderful women in the focus group who did the exercises, followed the food plan, and gave us helpful feedback: Ruth, Judy, Judith, Dianne, Jane, Batya, Sarah, Nancy, Therese, and Alexandra. For sharing their personal stories, I'm grateful to the women in the focus group, as well as to Susan, Isabel, Martha, Lillian, Diana, Bobbie, Deborah, Denise, Regina, Pat, Sue, Flora, Jill, and Verna.

Thank you to Dorothy Barron, Susan Zellman-Rohrer, Leslie Abad, Felina Mucha-Kangas, Cora Thompson, Carolyn Resendes, Mary Ellen Alonso, Judy Deemys, Yukiyo Iida, and Claudia Wiatr for their assistance with the illustrations and various aspects of the book.

Finally, I want to thank my family and friends for their great encouragement with this project. I especially want to thank my husband, Kin, and my children, Mason, Eliza, and Alexandra, for their continuous love, patience, and support.

The *Strong Women Stay Slim* program of diet and exercise is based on extensive scientific research. The book contains detailed instructions and safety cautions—I urge you to read them carefully. If you are under a physician's care for a medical condition, discuss this program with him or her before you start. Remember that regular medical checkups are essential to a healthy lifestyle. No book can possibly replace the services of a health care provider who knows you personally.

I

WEIGHING THE
SCIENTIFIC EVIDENCE

PUTTING NEW MUSCLE

INTO WEIGHT LOSS

From my teens through my twenties, I was always struggling with the same twenty pounds. I didn't eat excessive amounts, but I ate the wrong foods—a lot of sweets. I managed to lose ten pounds through excessive aerobic exercise: I'd go to step class for an hour, then spend forty-five minutes on a stair climber. But even that stopped working when I was in my early thirties.

I was determined to lose ten more pounds, and I wanted to eat better. So a year and a half ago I began to follow a flexible, healthy diet that I could adapt to my lifestyle. In two months I lost four pounds, and I stopped stressing out about food. Then I started strength training, and it made all the difference! I lost that last six pounds, and my figure changed. I'd been pear-shaped— my tops were size 10, but my bottoms were size 12 or 14. Now I can wear size 10 suits. My strength has increased tenfold. I got married a few months ago, and my husband was amazed by what I could lift when we were moving into our new home. He said, "I can't believe how strong you are!"

— Susan

◆ ◆ ◆

I went through some difficult changes in my life when I turned 40, and gained about forty pounds. I avoided looking in the mirror— I wore huge tanks and covered myself up. Then my picture was in the local newspaper. I was appalled; I didn't recognize myself. I joined a weight-loss class at my HMO and started doing aerobics, but I was having pain in my knees and hips. It hadn't occurred to me to add strength training until I saw an article about the re- search at Tufts. I decided to try it.

The results have been a dream come true. I've lost the weight. I feel so much younger; I have so much more energy. I can do things I didn't think were possible. I used to run—I love how it makes me feel. But I'd written that off when I was 35, because my orthopedist said, "Don't do it if it makes your knees and hips hurt." Now I can run every other day for an hour. Because I feel stronger physically, I feel like a stronger person from a psychologi- cal standpoint. My picture was in the paper again recently, and I was quite pleased!
— Isabel

◆ ◆ ◆

'm a scientist at the Jean Mayer USDA Human Nutrition Research Center on Aging at Tufts University. For the past ten years, our laboratory has studied the health benefits of strength training. My particular research has shown that strengthening exercise can prevent the loss of muscle and bone that debilitates so many women later in life. Along the way, I've become in- creasingly excited by another discovery: that strength training is also a re- markably effective aid to weight loss.

You may have read my first book, *Strong Women Stay Young*, which ex- plains the benefits of weight lifting. The book was based on my research, pub- lished in the *Journal of the American Medical Association (JAMA)*, showing that strengthening exercise not only makes women stronger, but also builds bone, improves balance and flexibility, and increases energy. I had recruited forty women who were at risk for muscle and bone loss: they were post- menopausal, sedentary, and not taking hormones. Before they started, I warned the volunteers that they'd have to avoid changes that could confuse our findings: for the next year they could *not* lose weight or begin aerobic exercise.

The women were very conscientious. But they changed anyway—they couldn't help it:

- ♦ Dorothy, who had been wearing size 16, was careful to maintain her weight. But after a few months of strength training, she noticed that her clothing was becoming loose. "I knew I needed a smaller size, so I bought 14s," she says. "Then I had to take them back because I needed 12s and sometimes 10s. My legs and hips became trimmer, and my arms got much more firm."

- ♦ Verna was shapelier, thanks to strength training. "My weight was never out of control, but there was fat in the wrong places," she says. "My inner thigh flab trimmed up, my upper arms got firmer, and I lost my tummy."

- ♦ Flora kept her promise not to start aerobics. But her new strength gave her so much extra energy that she took up ballroom dancing. Says Flora, "My girlfriend kept asking me to come with her, but I used to think the muscles in my calves would bother me. Now I can dance all night."

While this project was going on, my colleagues and I began a pilot study to see if strength training could prevent muscle and bone loss in another especially vulnerable group: women who were losing weight. Many women are shocked to learn that this is an at-risk category. They assume that when they lose weight, the only thing their body burns up is unwanted excess fat. Until recently that's what doctors and scientists believed too. But researchers have taken a closer look and discovered something disturbing: **When women diet, at least 25 to 30 percent of the weight they shed isn't fat, but water, muscle, bone, and other lean tissue.** This is true no matter how much protein and calcium their food plan includes. And the faster they lose weight, the larger the proportion that isn't fat.

I had been greatly encouraged by research from the University of Michigan showing that strength training could help women preserve muscle while they lost weight, and I wanted to explore this further. For our pilot study, my colleagues and I put ten overweight women on individually customized food plans designed for slow but steady weight loss. Half of them came to our laboratory twice a week and did strength training; the others just followed the diet.

Our diet-only volunteers lost an average of 13.0 pounds during the study. The women who strength trained lost about the same amount—13.2 pounds. But the scale didn't tell the whole story. A dramatic difference emerged when we looked at body composition. Women in the diet-only group had lost an average 2.8 pounds of lean tissue—mainly muscle—along with the fat. In contrast, the women who'd done strength training actually *gained* 1.4 pounds of lean tissue. So every ounce they lost was fat. Indeed, since the new muscle replaced fat, their total fat loss was 14.6 pounds. They lost 44 percent more fat than the diet-only group.

Our volunteers were thrilled to find an exercise at which they could excel. They became stronger, fitter, healthier, much more physically active—and were filled with self-confidence. Pat, who lost twenty-nine pounds, says:

> *Strength training helped the weight loss a lot. My metabolic rate went up, so I can eat more. I wear a smaller size than if I'd just lost weight and didn't build muscle. My doctor was very happy because my cholesterol and blood pressure went down. I have so much more energy—I feel invigorated. It gives you more self-esteem, a more positive feeling about anything you want to do.*

After *Strong Women Stay Young* was published, I received hundreds of letters, faxes, phone calls, and e-mail messages from readers all over the world. Many of these women found, to their great delight, that strength training had helped them lose weight. Inches, as well as pounds, had vanished. They looked better, felt healthier. Becoming strong had boosted their energy and vitality. Letter after letter spoke of new happiness and self-confidence.

- ◆ Diana: *I've only lost ten pounds, but people are saying, "You are losing so fast!"*

- ◆ Bobbie: *I'm now 42, but I feel like I'm in my twenties! Two years ago I was ten pounds heavier, had constant back pain, and felt slightly depressed. I was walking four miles a day, and thought this was all I should be doing. Then I started weight training, and everything changed. I wish I had discovered this*

*ten years ago. I feel so good! I ski, and I do in-line skating—
they were easy to master once I was strong.*

Along with the progress reports came questions:

*Should I be doing aerobics too—and if so, how much?
What food should I eat?
Do I need to take a vitamin supplement if I'm losing weight?*

I have the great privilege to work at Tufts University, along with dozens of other scientists involved in exciting new research on nutrition, exercise, and health. I discussed the readers' concerns with my colleagues, as well as with some of the many experts from other institutions who visit our laboratories to exchange information. I began to realize how much different specialists have learned about what works for healthy long-term weight loss. What was needed, I became convinced, was a comprehensive program that would pull together the essential pieces. I wanted to combine new findings about strength training with up-to-date information on nutrition and physical activity. My aim was to come up with a practical program that would not only help women lose weight permanently, but would also become the foundation for a long, healthy, vibrant life. That's why I decided to write *Strong Women Stay Slim.*

THE DESPERATE STRUGGLE

So many women are battling to lose weight—yet they keep getting heavier and heavier. Since 1980 the prevalence of overweight in American women has jumped by nearly 10 percent, according to the U.S. Department of Health and Human Services. We don't need government statistics to see the changes as we get older. One woman in five is overweight in her twenties. The problem intensifies during the later reproductive years: more than a third of women age 30 to 49 weigh too much. But the numbers really soar at menopause. An astonishing 52 percent of women in their fifties are overweight.

We all know that excess weight endangers health. Overweight triples the normal risk for heart disease and stroke, contributes to diabetes, and has even been linked to cancer. Dr. C. Everett Koop, the former U.S. Surgeon General, estimates that 300,000 Americans die from overweight-related causes each year! And millions of heavy women suffer from associated medical conditions that diminish the quality of their lives—from heartburn, to joint pain, to infertility. The burden is emotional as well. Many women are caught in a sad vicious circle: feeling depressed about their weight, seeking consolation in food, gaining more weight, and feeling even worse.

In desperation, some turn to risky medications and fad diets. But it's actually healthier to remain heavy than to lose weight the wrong way. I'm not just talking about the obvious dangers, like life-threatening side effects from drugs or nutritional deficiencies from unbalanced diets. Even the standard "sensible" advice—to eat 1000 to 1200 calories a day—puts women at risk because they lose so much lean tissue along with fat.

Preserving muscle and bone is vitally important for women. We start out with a lot less muscle and bone than men do, so we have a narrower margin of safety. Yet we live longer, so we're much more likely to reach an age where our lives are severely limited by muscular weakness or fragile bones.

But there's a much more immediate reason to be concerned about the loss of lean tissue: the less muscle you have, the harder it is to lose weight and to maintain the loss. Muscle is metabolically active; body fat isn't. So the smaller the proportion of lean tissue in your body, the lower your metabolic rate. To make matters worse, when you lose muscle, you become weaker and have less energy. Consequently you're likely to burn fewer calories through physical activity. If you've ever hit a long plateau during a diet and remained stuck at the same weight despite all your efforts, this could be a reason.

The kind of dieting that leads to muscle loss also sabotages metabolism in another way: by cutting calories too drastically. Nature cleverly designed the human body so we could survive famine. If you put yourself on starvation rations—and for some women even 1200 calories a day is starving—you trigger hormonal shifts that help the body conserve calories instead of burning them. But when you're trying to lose weight, that's the last thing you want! Between the starvation effect and muscle loss, **the wrong diet can reduce your metabolic rate by up to 30 percent.**

These metabolic changes help explain the all-too-common phenomenon of "yo-yo" dieting: a woman manages to lose weight—but in the process she undermines herself by depressing her metabolism. Maintaining the loss is a losing battle. She's ravenous all the time; her energy disappears. Eventually she gives in to her hunger and quickly regains.

After one of these discouraging cycles, a woman might console herself with the thought that she's no worse off than when she started her diet. Unfortunately, that's not true. The weight she lost was partly lean tissue, but nearly everything she regained is fat. Because she has less muscle now, it's going to be harder than ever to lose. What's more, repeated bouts of yo-yo dieting increase her risk for heart disease and stroke.

Once scientists and doctors understood the key role of lean tissue in metabolism, they began looking for ways that people could conserve muscle while shedding pounds. The answer turned out to be very simple: strengthening exercise.

THE FAT-FIGHTING POWER OF STRENGTH TRAINING

With strength training, you don't merely lose weight—you give yourself the leaner, healthier body of someone who's naturally slim. The benefits start with muscle and metabolism, but they go even further.

Here's how strength training helps you lose weight forever:

PRESERVES MUSCLE AND BONE AS YOU SHED FAT

I've already explained that women usually lose muscle when they diet. Another disturbing finding, of particular concern to women: at least seven well-controlled studies have shown that when you diet and lose weight, you lose bone too. A 1994 study done at the Queens Medical Centre in Nottingham, England, studied premenopausal women who dieted for three months. Even though they followed a sensible food plan for modest weight loss (the average was just 7.5 pounds), they lost 1 percent of their bone mass. That's an alarming change for so short a period in women under age 50, who normally lose no more than half a percent in an entire year.

We know that strength training can preserve muscle when women are losing weight, and we think that it may help prevent bone loss as well. Several investigators currently are examining this question, and I look forward to seeing their results.

◆ REVS UP YOUR METABOLISM

Have you ever noticed that your male friends and relatives can eat much more than you do without gaining weight? Men really do have a metabolic advantage. But the explanation isn't their hormones, it's their muscles.

Strength training gives your metabolism a boost. You burn calories when you strength train—and you also burn more calories throughout the day when you have more lean tissue. In a study by Wayne Campbell, Ph.D., in our laboratory, which was published in the *American Journal of Clinical Nutrition,* the combined difference amounted to about 15 percent. That translates into an extra 300 calories per day for the average woman.

◆ FIRMS AND TIGHTENS, SO YOU LOOK TRIMMER

A pound of fat is bulkier than a pound of muscle. So if your weight loss is almost all fat, you'll look trimmer than if you lose lean tissue too. The women in my *JAMA* study all agreed not to lose weight. Nevertheless, many of them dropped one to three sizes because their bodies were more toned.

Nancy, one of the women in the group that tested the program in this book, reported:

> *The other day I needed a dress for a wedding. My teenage daughter had a navy sheath that was perfect. But I had been size 14 going on size 16, and this was size 12. Also, the dress didn't have sleeves, and I'd never worn anything sleeveless because my arms were always too flabby. I tried it on anyway. My daughter said, "It looks great—your arms aren't flabby at all!" So that's what I wore.*

◆ EASES YOU INTO A MORE PHYSICALLY ACTIVE LIFESTYLE

Becoming more active is not only a tremendous help to weight loss—it's also the key to staying slim. First, you burn extra calories when you move. Second, your metabolism remains slightly elevated for several hours after exercise. Third, there's evidence that being active helps tame your appetite. Moreover, an active lifestyle conditions your heart and lungs, making you fitter and healthier.

The problem is that many overweight women don't enjoy physical activity—and for good reason. Understandably, they feel self-conscious about pulling on spandex leggings and joining an exercise class. Even walking has little appeal for someone who's out of shape, especially if her joints ache and she becomes winded in a few minutes.

Strength training makes all the difference. The stronger your muscles, the easier it is to get moving. All the women in my *JAMA* study, as I've mentioned, previously were sedentary and had actually been directed *not* to begin an exercise program. Nevertheless, these revitalized women spontaneously began walking more, climbing more steps, and selecting more active leisure activities like dancing, hiking, and gardening. When we added it all up, after a year of strength training they had become 27 percent more active! We've now seen similar results in three other studies.

◆ MAKES YOU HEALTHIER

You've heard about weight-loss methods that carry alarming risks—surgery that could shorten your life, pills that might damage your heart. Strength training is different. Instead of risks and side effects, it offers impressive health *advantages*. All women benefit from increased strength. Women over age 40 gain even more, because strength training reverses age-related muscle and bone loss; it even improves balance and flexibility. Indeed, as I'll explain in Chapter 3, strength training is one of the most effective ways to combat osteoporosis and the frailty too often associated with aging.

◆　◆　◆

When I was 36, I had a blood clot in my leg. I'm 48 now, and I'm looking toward menopause. I know I'm not a candidate for estrogen therapy. Strength training is a great alternative.
— *Martha*

◆　◆　◆

◆ HELPS YOU FEEL GOOD ABOUT YOURSELF

When I work with women who are strength training, some of the most significant changes I see are emotional. Physical strength is something that women rarely expect of themselves. But when a woman becomes strong, her self-confidence and self-esteem soar. The effect is especially powerful for women who are overweight and sedentary.

Excess weight is a handicap for many forms of exercise—but not for strength training. Indeed, very heavy women are often quite strong. It's always a special joy to watch an overweight woman—someone who has never succeeded at any physical activity in her entire life—discover that she's not merely capable of lifting weights but actually good at it! Her whole view of herself is transformed.

Over and over, I've seen strength training open the door for weight loss. Dianne, one of the women in the group that helped me refine the program for this book, isn't sure exactly how much she weighed when she started because her scale doesn't register above 300 pounds. "I figure it was about 340," she says. Aerobic exercise was out of the question for her—even five minutes of walking left her winded and made her legs ache unbearably. "I wanted to exercise, but how could I? I was a ball of jelly," says Dianne. "Then I read about strength training. Boing! A light went off in my head. Here was something that would bring me to a point where I could be more active."

Dianne became the star of our test group, rapidly graduating from 3-pound dumbbells, to 5-pound, then 8-, 10-, and even 15-pound dumbbells for some exercises. Other changes followed. "Strength training gave me an overall sense of wellness, and it snowballed," says Dianne. "I started to eat better within two weeks. I could see myself getting more involved in my own life, being better to myself. I became more active in little ways—instead of sending my daughter upstairs to get my earrings or my watch, I'd go myself. I frequently parked at the far end of parking lots."

By the end of ten weeks, Dianne had lost more than thirty-five pounds—and she glowed with vitality. The woman who could barely manage a five-minute walk when she started had joined a gym and was regularly walking thirty minutes on a treadmill. Says Dianne, "It's been a great uplift—I feel so much more positive." I'm thrilled with Dianne's progress so far and look forward to watching her continue.

THE *STRONG WOMEN STAY SLIM* PROGRAM

The *Strong Women Stay Slim* program combines the power of strength training with nutritious eating and an active lifestyle. It's not just a weight-loss program; it's a way to become healthier for a lifetime.

EXERCISE YOU CAN DO

Regardless how much you weigh, you can become active and fit. Instead of starting with aerobic exercise, this program begins with strength training. There's no huffing and puffing, no special clothes, no getting down on the floor (and struggling to get up again). You'll love the quick results you get with strength training. What a confidence booster!

If you've been sedentary, you'll systematically increase your activity in your third week on the program. By then you'll be stronger, so moving will be easier and more fun. Over the next eight weeks you'll slowly build up strength and endurance—never pushing yourself too far or too fast—until, by the tenth week, you'll join the 25 percent of American adults who get at least thirty minutes of moderate physical activity three or more times a week.

A DIET THAT'S REALISTIC

Most programs put all overweight women on the same 1000- to 1200-calorie diet. But one diet plan does *not* fit all. For many, a 1200-calorie diet is self-defeating because it cuts food intake too drastically. They try to comply, but hunger usually wins. The *Strong Women Stay Slim* program has 1200-, 1600-, and 2000-calorie plans, so it adjusts for everyone. You'll learn how to **eat to the limit**—to adjust your intake so you continue to lose, while eating as much healthy food as possible.

Let's face it: if you're trying to lose weight, you can't eat as much as you want of whatever you want. But if deprivation has kept you from succeeding in the past, I can offer you two important promises:

- **First, you can eat the foods you love.** There are no forbidden foods on this program. You can have a slice of chocolate cake on your birthday; you can order barbecued ribs at your favorite restaurant.

◆ **Second, you never need to be hungry.** In addition to ample meals and snacks, you can have almost unlimited amounts of certain filling and nutritious foods.

A VIBRANT NEW LIFESTYLE

Of course, you want to lose weight to improve your appearance. But I hope you're also concerned about your health. Some weight-reduction measures force you to chose between looking good and feeling good, but not this one. Instead of worrisome side effects, this program offers added *benefits*—increased vitality and strength, improved mood and sleep, better balance and flexibility, plus reduced risk of heart disease, diabetes, cancer, arthritis, and other debilitating conditions.

◆ ◆ ◆

I'm not just happy about the weight loss; I'm happy about how *I'm losing weight. I love being strong. I like knowing that my diet is healthy and that I'm getting regular aerobic exercise. My husband keeps telling me how proud he is of what I'm doing.*
    — Alexandra

◆ ◆ ◆

TEN WEEKS TO A NEW YOU

The *Strong Women Stay Slim* program lets you bypass the dangers and deprivation of quick-weight-loss programs. You lose weight steadily, at the sensible rate that doctors recommend—one-half pound to two pounds a week. But thanks to strength training, you'll see *results* just as quickly as with risky, counterproductive quick-loss programs. As you trade fat for muscle (which is more compact), you'll look trimmer. You'll also see fast results in the form of increased energy and strength. Most women experience thrilling improvements in less than a month.

Here's where you'll be at the end of ten weeks:

- **If you needed to lose five to ten pounds,** you will have reached this goal by losing half a pound to a pound per week over the entire ten-week period. You may have been battling that same five or ten pounds for years! Now, thanks to weight loss and exercise, you should be shapelier as well as slimmer. And the weight is gone for good.

- **If you needed to lose between ten and fifty pounds,** you will have lost about ten pounds. I realize that may not sound like much if you're used to the quick results of fad diets. But because you've also been doing strength training and aerobic exercise, you'll probably look much more than ten pounds slimmer. More important, this time you won't have to put up with inconvenient (and unnecessary) food restrictions or go hungry. Instead, you'll be following a sensible plan that will let you lose the remaining weight and stay slim and healthy for the rest of your life.

- **If you need to lose more than fifty pounds,** you'll shed ten to twenty pounds during the first ten weeks—a significant start. Adding to this loss will be the slimming effects of your fitness program. For the first time you'll have a food plan that doesn't starve you, and exercise that allows you to succeed. I'm sure you'll be brimming with self-confidence. Just keep going, and your weight loss will continue. You're establishing the lifestyle that will keep the weight off forever.

You can expect other changes, regardless of where you started:

- You'll feel stronger and more capable physically; you'll have much more energy.

- You'll sleep better at night.

- Your chronic aches and pains may disappear.

- Your self-esteem will increase; you'll feel happier. You'll look in the mirror and like what you see.

Not visible but vitally important are the improvements to your cardiovascular system, your muscles, your bones, and your balance.

◆ ◆ ◆

In the past when I went on a diet, I would try to motivate myself by thinking about reaching my ideal size. But the task seemed overwhelming. Eventually I'd say to myself, "Forget it—I'll never get there." This time I'm getting immediate gratification, and that keeps me going. My strength and energy increased right away; my stress level is way down. I'm out of bed before the alarm goes off. And people are starting to comment on how much better I look.
—*Ruth*

◆ ◆ ◆

WHAT THIS BOOK PROVIDES

You're about to start a program that will change how you live. You'll lose weight safely and permanently. This book will tell you everything you need to know:

◆ UP-TO-THE-MINUTE SCIENTIFIC INFORMATION

The more you know, the more motivated you will be.

◆ Chapter 2 explains what it takes to control appetite and get your metabolism on your side. You'll learn why some diets fail—and why this one will work.

◆ Chapter 3 explains exactly how strength training—along with a more active lifestyle—promotes weight loss, tightens and trims your figure, and offers significant health benefits. Exercise not only helps you look and feel better right now, it also reduces your long-term risk for almost all major chronic diseases. No medication can match it.

♦ Chapter 4 explains how a healthy diet helps you live slimmer as well as longer. Good nutrition tames hunger and cravings, so you lose weight more easily and keep it off.

DETAILED STEP-BY-STEP INSTRUCTIONS

I'll give you complete directions, and tell you how to adapt this program to your particular needs.

♦ Chapter 7 gives you a strength-training program—six basic moves designed for weight loss, plus optional supplemental exercises you can add later.

♦ Chapter 8 provides directions for becoming more active, with a self-test that ensures you get on the right track and progress safely.

♦ Chapter 9 presents the food plan, with basic instructions and menus that can be adapted to any lifestyle.

♦ Chapter 10 will help you put everything together, so you're on your way.

♦ Chapter 12 answers common questions about the program.

MOTIVATIONAL SAVVY

It's not easy to make changes in your life, even when you know they're important. In our research at Tufts, where we need to follow volunteers for many months, we've worked very hard to learn how to motivate participants. I'm very proud of the fact that our dropout rates are among the lowest reported in the medical literature. Even if you're not coming into our labs every week, what we've learned can work for you.

♦ Chapter 5 draws upon sports psychology to explain the mental secrets of successful weight loss.

♦ Chapter 6 helps you decide what you should weigh—the number may surprise you.

- ◆ Chapter 11 will help you keep yourself on track and overcome any obstacles you may encounter.

◆ TEN DAYS OF INNOVATIVE MENUS AND RECIPES BASED ON THE FOOD PLAN

To get you off to a good start, I asked renowned cookbook author Steven Raichlen to prepare menus and recipes. As the recipes came in, I had great fun trying them. You'll be delighted—as my family and I were—to see how well you can eat on this plan.

You are about to start a program that will change your life forever. You're taking charge, and doing something wonderful for yourself. Expect a very positive experience, right from the start.

THE SURPRISING

REASON THAT

WOMEN GAIN

After my daughter was born, I couldn't lose weight. I started to think about diet pills, even though I knew that was a dangerous road. I tried a commercial diet organization for a while, but it was expensive. Besides, I don't like to be told what I can and can't eat.
— *Therese*

◆   ◆   ◆

You're smart, you're disciplined about work—yet you can't seem to lose weight. Or maybe you're able to lose (you've done it dozens of times), but you can't keep the weight off. You know it's not just a matter of willpower, because you have ample willpower in other areas of your life. The situation is all the more frustrating because weight loss sounds simple: *Just eat less.* You've probably gotten this well-meant advice from friends and relatives. You may have told yourself the same thing. But you don't know why it's so difficult.

In fact, weight loss isn't simple at all. Intricate and powerful systems in our bodies regulate both appetite and metabolism in what seems like a conspiracy to keep us at our present weight. To make matters worse, stringent dieting actually exacerbates the situation by slowing metabolism and leaving the appetite unsatisfied. Fortunately, solutions are starting to emerge—and it's becoming increasingly clear that "Just eat less" isn't the answer.

THE DELICATE BALANCE

My work gives me the opportunity to talk with women of all ages and sizes about their weight problems. Some have been heavy all their lives; others are trying to get rid of the excess from their last pregnancy, or they're worried about gaining during menopause. These women are very different from each other, but many of them tell me the same thing:

I can't seem to lose weight, but I really don't eat that much.

And I respond: *I know you're right!*

Usually they're very surprised—other people always assume they overeat. But that's often not the problem.

Whether you gain or lose weight depends on your **energy balance**—how much food energy you burn compared to how much you consume. This energy is measured in **calories**. We sometimes talk about calories as if they were tiny pellets crammed into a dish of ice cream or a portion of steak. In fact, a calorie is a measurement unit, the amount of energy required to raise the temperature of 1 gram of water by 1 degree Celsius. The word comes from the Latin "calor," which means heat.

Food energy—calories—is what keeps our bodies alive and functioning. To maintain a consistent weight, our caloric intake must equal caloric output. If we eat more than we burn, the excess is stored as body fat. All of us have days when we go way over on intake, but the equation doesn't have to balance every single day so long as things generally come out even. I always feel bad when I hear a woman berating herself for enjoying good food at a party. Special events are rarely responsible for weight problems. Rather, the pounds accumulate because of *small but consistent* imbalances. Just 50 calories a day of extra intake or insufficient caloric expenditure adds up to five pounds a year. When a woman tells me that creeping weight gain has left her fifty pounds heavier than she was ten years ago, I know that 50 calories a day could account for it. Those dramatic government statistics about the increasing prevalence of overweight in women, which I mentioned in Chapter 1, reflect very small imbalances, not rampant gluttony.

When you hear about a 50-calorie excess, you might automatically think of food—a woman could get 50 extra calories from half an apple or a few crackers, or simply by adding cream and sugar to a cup of coffee. Until recently experts also focused mostly on the intake side of the energy balance equation. But decades ago a different hypothesis was proposed by the late Jean Mayer, Ph.D., the famous nutritionist for whom our Tufts research center is named. Dr. Mayer believed that overweight usually was caused *not* by excessive caloric intake, but by insufficient caloric expenditure—the other side of the equation. When he first proposed this idea, back in the 1950s, most nutritionists thought he was way off base. Since then, accumulated evidence has proven that he was absolutely right:

The surprising reason that women gain is that they're burning too few calories.

We now know that most women aren't getting heavier because they eat more. Moreover, it doesn't take much of a discrepancy to cause significant weight gain over time. But the balance can just as easily be tipped in the other direction. Weight loss doesn't require stringent dieting or grueling exercise. Small but consistent changes can produce a remarkable difference—and strength training makes it easy.

IS YOUR METABOLISM WORKING AGAINST YOU?

My husband eats whatever he wants—fried chicken, premium ice cream, you name it—and he can still fit into pants he bought twenty years ago. How come I gain weight if I so much as look at a potato chip? It's not fair!

◆　◆　◆

I get questions like this all the time. So many women look around and are baffled to see other people eating more but weighing less. They wonder if there's something wrong with them. Could it be their genes, or maybe a thyroid problem? Is it just an inevitable consequence of being a woman or of getting older? Yes, all of these factors can play a role, and they help explain why weight loss is so difficult.

The calories we burn fall into three categories:

- **Basal metabolism**—the energy our body needs to remain alive—accounts for 50 to 75 percent of our daily caloric expenditure.

- **Digestion**—we use about 10 percent of the calories we consume to process food.

- **Physical activity**—15 to 40 percent of our caloric expenditure is used for activities above the basal metabolic baseline.

As you'll see, nature may indeed be working against you. Even so, there's a great deal you can do to rev up your metabolism.

Basal Metabolism

Your basal metabolic rate (BMR) is the energy you consume when you're awake but not using any calories to move. In the laboratory we measure it first thing in the morning, before our volunteers get out of bed. Basal metabolism reflects all the work your body does to sustain life: the beating of your heart, the activities of all your other organs, the functioning of your brain, temperature regulation, and the tiny repairs that keep your muscles and bones in working order.

Metabolism, as many women suspect, is not fair. Your genetic heritage helps determine your metabolic rate, as well as the shape of your body. However, the lifestyle you picked up from your parents contributes too—and that part can be altered. Men really do have an advantage, as I'll explain below. It's also true that our basal metabolic rate typically decreases as we get older. But as you'll see, behind the sex and age differences are differences in body composition and activity. Indeed, the single most important factor in determining BMR is the amount of lean tissue in our body. This is very good news because it means **we can increase our basal metabolic rate by 15 percent or more, simply by building muscle and becoming more active.**

Why It's Easier for Men

A woman of average weight has a basal metabolic rate of about 1300 calories, but the average normal-weight man has an BMR of about 1700 calo-

How to Estimate Your Basal Metabolic Rate

Precise measurement of the basal metabolic rate requires elaborate scientific equipment. However, you can use the following equation, called the Harris-Benedict formula, to make an estimate. This version is calibrated for women; though it takes weight, height, and age into account, other factors—especially the amount of lean tissue in your body—are also very important:

4.4 × [weight in pounds] + 4.7 × [height in inches] - 4.7 [age in years] + 655.

Here's how to do the calculation:

Step 1: Multiply your weight in pounds by 4.4 _____\
Step 2: Multiply your height in inches by 4.7 _____\
Step 3: Add answers from Step 1 and Step 2 _____\
Step 4: Multiply your age in years by 4.7 _____\
Step 5: Subtract Step 4 answer from Step 3 _____\
Step 6: Add 655 to the answer from Step 5 _____\

If your weight is normal or slightly above normal, the answer in Step 6 is a good approximation of your BMR—the number of calories you burn each day simply by being alive. If you're very overweight, this will slightly overestimate your BMR by 10 to 15 percent.

Example: Linda weighs 173 pounds; she's 5 feet 5 inches (65 inches) tall, and 38 years old.

Step 1: Multiply your weight in pounds by 4.4	761
Step 2: Multiply your height in inches by 4.7	306
Step 3: Add answers from Step 1 and Step 2	1067
Step 4: Multiply your age in years by 4.7	179
Step 5: Subtract Step 4 answer from Step 3	888
Step 6: Add 655 to the answer from Step 5	1543

Linda's BMR is 1,543 calories.

ries—a 400-calorie advantage! Hormones explain some of it, but not much. Far more important is the difference in their body composition. He weighs 160 pounds; she weighs 125 pounds. He's leaner as well as heavier, with 12 percent body fat to her 20 percent. So his metabolism is driven by 140 pounds of lean tissue, compared to just 100 pounds for her.

In other words, it's not his testosterone, it's his muscles.

What Happens as We Get Older

If you haven't yet experienced this change for yourself, you've probably heard your older women friends and relatives complain about it:

I'm not eating any differently, but I'm gaining weight.
I can't have dessert anymore.

The explanation is very simple: as we age, we usually burn fewer calories. The basal metabolic rate of an average 60-year-old is about 200 calories a day lower than the BMR of a typical 30-year-old. Most of the difference can be explained by body composition. Starting around age 40, most women lose about a third of a pound of muscle each year (and gain at least that much body fat); they also lose smaller amounts of bone. These changes accelerate at perimenopause and during early menopause. At this time of her life, a woman can lose five pounds of muscle in just five years—unless she compensates with strengthening exercise.

Physical Activity Kick-Starts the Engine

We've known for a long time that exercise can compensate for the age-related decline in basal metabolism. Intriguing new research suggests that physical activity does even more: it can actually halt this change.

Investigators at the University of Colorado compared sedentary and active postmenopausal women age 50 to 72 with women age 21 to 35. The older women who were sedentary showed the expected decrease in BMR compared with their younger counterparts. But *older women who were physically active had the same BMRs on average as active women half their age!*

Overly Stringent Dieting Undermines Metabolism

Our bodies seem to think we're still living on the prehistoric savanna, where drought might strike or the hunting might be bad, instead of around the corner from a supermarket. When a woman cuts calories too drastically, her body has no idea she's trying to lose weight—so her thyroid gland leaps into action to protect her from starvation.

The thyroid gland, a butterfly-shaped organ located in the neck, regulates metabolism by secreting a hormone called thyroxine. The amount you secrete is influenced by what you eat. If you consume fewer calories than your body burns, your thyroid tries to compensate by cutting back on thyroxine: your metabolism slows down and you feel sluggish, so you don't move around as much. These are *not* abnormalities—your thyroid is just doing its job and trying to conserve body tissue. Usually the effect is too small to be noticed. However, it becomes significant if a woman fasts or follows a very low-calorie diet. Such extremes can cause her BMR to plummet by as much as 30 percent. That's why it's so important to eat enough when you're trying to lose weight.

This perfectly normal thyroid response should not be confused with thyroid disorders that affect weight. Some women gain because their thyroid glands are underactive, a condition called **hypothyroidism**. Symptoms include not only sluggish metabolism, but also fatigue, depression, dry skin, constipation, and sensitivity to cold. Though hypothyroidism is uncommon, even in overweight women, anyone who suspects she might have this problem can take a simple blood test to find out for sure. The condition is readily treated with synthetic thyroid hormone.

FOOD HELPS YOU BURN CALORIES

It takes calories to burn calories. About 10 percent of your daily caloric intake is used to process that food. In other words, if you consume about 2000 calories a day, approximately 200 calories are burned just for digestion. Though this is an important part of the energy balance equation, you can't do much to change it. *There's no scientific evidence that particular combinations of foods will help you burn more calories.* Some foods—including high-fiber grains, protein foods, fruits, and vegetables—do require extra calories to digest. However, the difference is insignificant.

THE SIMPLEST WAY TO USE EXTRA CALORIES: PHYSICAL ACTIVITY

Physical activity is the part of caloric expenditure that varies the most from person to person, and it's also the easiest to modify. Any woman can significantly increase the number of calories she burns through activity.

Remember, it doesn't take much: I've already explained that for many women, the difference between slim and heavy is as little as 50 calories a day. Also, I'm not just talking about those activities we think of as exercise, like jogging around a track or taking a step-aerobics class. *All* activity counts.

Let me use myself as an example. I have a hearty appetite and eat about 2200 calories a day, yet I never gain weight. There's nothing magical about my metabolism. In fact, because I'm petite, my basal metabolic rate is slightly lower than average—only about 1280 calories a day. My body uses another 10 percent of my intake, around 220 calories a day, for digestion.

What about the remaining 700 calories? If I were sedentary, I'd burn only about 300 extra calories a day; unless I cut way back on food, I'd gain weight. But because I'm physically active, I use up the entire 700 calories, and my weight remains the same.

I strength train twice a week; I also make a point of getting at least forty-five minutes of aerobic exercise three or more times a week. That might sound like a lot of exercise, but if you add it all up, it averages out to only about 100 calories per day. What keeps my weight stable is all the rest of my physical activity: walking whenever possible instead of taking the car or bus, moving around the room when I talk on the phone instead of sitting in a chair, climbing stairs, playing active games with my children.

Modern conveniences have pushed physical activity out of our lives. We put telephone extensions all over the house so we don't need to walk from room to room; we toss laundry into the washing machine instead of laboring over a sink; we cut the grass with an electric mower instead of the human-powered kind. These are trivial changes—but they add up. In fact, they may explain most of the collective weight gain Americans have experienced over the past several decades. I'm not suggesting you return to the scrub board! But the more active you become, the higher your metabolism will be.

Because overweight makes moving harder, women often pick up sedentary habits along with extra pounds: they use the remote instead of getting up to change channels; they ask a child to fetch the mail. These patterns can be subtle. One fascinating study, done long ago by Dr. Jean Mayer and colleagues, filmed heavy and normal girls as they played tennis, then analyzed their moves. The normal-weight youngsters were in constant motion during the game, but their overweight counterparts hardly budged except when hitting the ball.

When women become stronger, they naturally become more active. At the end of a year of strength training, the women in my *JAMA* study were an astonishing 27 percent more active, despite having been asked not to do additional exercise. When you begin strength training, you'll experience the same vitalizing change. I hope you'll also make a conscious effort to build more physical activity into your daily life—I'll give you lots of specific suggestions in Chapter 8. Here's a special incentive: the more you weigh, the more calories you'll burn when you get active. For instance, a 115-pound woman might use up about 45 calories during a brisk ten-minute walk. But a 200-pound woman who took exactly the same walk would burn about 75 calories—it takes extra energy to move more weight.

FAT ISN'T ALL BAD!

Our bodies are *supposed* to contain some fat. Here's what it does for us:

- **Provides an energy reserve**—Our fat stores are nature's way of enabling us to withstand starvation.

- **Cushions our bodies**—Vital organs, like the kidneys, liver, and intestines, are padded with a protective layer of fat.

- **Acts as insulation**—The layer of fat just under your skin helps keep you warm in the winter. (Of course, if you have too much fat, you'll get overheated in the summer.)

- **Synthesizes estrogen and other hormones**—These hormones are necessary for many processes in the body.

♦ ♦ ♦

I live in a two-story house with a basement, and I used to avoid going up and down the steps—this was very efficient, but not very smart since I want to use up more calories. A couple of weeks ago

I decided to give myself points for climbing stairs. I put an index card and pencil at the top of the stairs, and every time I come up-stairs, I get a point. It worked! When I started, I made five to ten trips a day; now I'm up to fifteen to twenty.
  — Alexandra

◆ ◆ ◆

How Women Get Hit with a Double Whammy

Once you understand the importance of basal metabolism and physical activity in the energy-balance equation, you can see why women are so vulnerable to weight problems at key times in their lives.

Postpartum Pounds

I'd always been slender, but things changed when I became preg-nant. During the first few months I felt nauseated and tired, and I discovered that sugar gave me relief. That's when I began using food for comfort. Also, my lifestyle became more sedentary, espe-cially after my second child was born. One day I woke up and re-alized that I weighed exactly what I'd weighed when I delivered my first baby—except I wasn't pregnant.
  — Martha

◆ ◆ ◆

A twenty-five- to thirty-five-pound weight gain is healthy during pregnancy. Extra fluid and the developing baby account for most of that; your body also accumulates fat reserves. After birth, some women quickly return to their usual weight. But for others, the extra pounds linger. The problem is of-ten compounded by all the changes motherhood brings.

Life with a new baby is hectic, but most women become more seden-tary in the postpartum months. At the same time that they're burning fewer calories through activity, other factors conspire to make them eat more: often they're not getting enough sleep, and research suggests that fatigue is easily confused with hunger. They're at home, where food is more readily available, and their usual meal patterns are disrupted. On top of everything else, new mothers often experience the mild form of depression known as the "baby blues," which can lead to the kind of "comfort eating" Martha describes. As the pounds mount up, unhappiness increases and the problem gets worse.

MONTHLY WEIGHT FLUCTUATIONS

Though we experience premenstrual changes regularly, it's hard not to be dismayed by them—the weight gain, the bloated feeling, and the voracious appetite. These problems are real, but fortunately only temporary. During the week to ten days before menstruation, women retain extra water and therefore put on several pounds. But they lose both liquid and weight by the time their period ends. Increased hunger does make women eat more when they're premenstrual. However, there's a corresponding rise in metabolic rate that usually compensates for it.

Women who take birth control pills often experience mild versions of premenstrual changes. Usually their body adapts in a month or two and the symptoms disappear. If you take oral contraceptives and have persistent weight problems, talk to your doctor. The solution could be as simple as another pill formulation.

Menopausal Metamorphosis

I'm a breast cancer survivor. Chemotherapy made me go into menopause, and I started to gain weight. Ten pounds hit me like a ton of bricks. Then another ten pounds crept on, until I weighed 165 pounds—more than I'd ever been in my life. I didn't feel well: my lower back hurt all the time; I didn't have a lot of energy. I tried skipping meals and starving myself, but I continued to gain.
    — *Nancy*

♦ ♦ ♦

I've already explained that women lose muscle when they start menopause. We know that hormonal changes are a contributing factor, but some of the loss is caused by decreased activity. Here too, a vicious circle begins: as women lose muscle, activity becomes more difficult. This leads to weight gain, which makes physical activity even harder. Meanwhile, lowered self-esteem and depression enter the picture, and may result in excess eating.

IS YOUR APPETITE OUT OF CONTROL?

Our appetite for food—like our instinctive need to breathe, drink, or sleep—is one of the biological mechanisms that keep us alive. But many women describe their hunger as an unreasonable and powerful force:

> *Half an hour after a big meal, I'm ravenous all over again.*
> *Once I start, I can't stop—it's like a truck rolling downhill with no brakes.*
> *When cravings hit, I can't think about anything else.*

The command center for our appetite is in a part of the brain called the **hypothalamus**. When we need food, the hypothalamus sends out signals that we're hungry. After we've eaten, the message changes and the hypothalamus announces that we're satiated. We don't yet fully understand all the processes involved, but we know that healthy eating and physical activity can help tame an unruly appetite.

Because hunger and satiety are so important to our well-being, nature has multiple mechanisms to deliver information to the hypothalamus:

STOMACH CONTRACTIONS

Our stomach contracts when it has been empty for a while, producing that tight feeling we call "hunger pangs." After we've eaten and our stomach is distended by food, we sense that we're full. This is the first signal of satiation, and it's one we can enhance with savvy food choices. If we drink plenty of fluids and select high-bulk but low-calorie foods (such as fiber-rich vegetables and whole grains), we'll feel full more quickly.

BLOOD SUGAR

During digestion, food is broken down into sugar, which enters the bloodstream for distribution to our cells. The hypothalamus monitors the amount of sugar in our blood. As the level goes up, the hypothalamus senses that we've eaten. Later, depletion of blood sugar signals that we need to eat again.

Nature probably intended us to consume small quantities of food throughout the day rather than getting most of our calories in just three meals. Our bodies don't always cope very well with the resulting "sugar spikes." Sometimes blood sugar levels shoot too high and then fall too rapidly, causing us to feel hungry when we've really had enough.

Wise food choices can help reduce these fluctuations in blood sugar, as I'll explain in Chapter 4. If your diet is high in complex carbohydrates, such as vegetables and whole grains, sugar is released more gradually and you feel full longer. Being strong and active also helps: the muscles act as a storage buffer for sugar, which means that levels in the blood are more consistent.

SIGNALS FROM THE INTESTINES

When food leaves the stomach and enters the small intestines, the intestinal lining releases several hormones. We know from experiments in animals that these hormones are powerful appetite suppressants. One of them, called **cholecystokinin** (CCK), also seems to contribute to the calming effect we experience after eating. CCK is especially responsive to fat in the diet.

It's useful to remember that some satiety signals aren't triggered until food is well along in the digestive process. That's one reason that it's so important to eat slowly, and to give your body a chance to realize it's been fed. Otherwise you may unwittingly overeat, then feel uncomfortably full later.

SEROTONIN AND OTHER CHEMICALS IN THE BRAIN

After we eat—particularly when we have foods rich in carbohydrates or dairy proteins—the brain releases chemicals, called neurotransmitters, that act on the nervous system. The best known of these neurotransmitters is **serotonin**, which not only influences hunger and satiety but also has a soothing effect. Many anti-depressant and anti-anxiety medications work by increasing serotonin levels or by making the brain more sensitive to existing supplies. If you reach for carbohydrate-rich food when you feel tense or unhappy, you're actually medicating yourself. Serotonin is very important, but it's just one of more than 500 neurotransmitters in the brain. Quite likely, others affect mood and appetite too. I expect we'll hear more about them as research continues.

Physical activity triggers the release of mood-affecting chemicals too. These hormones, called endorphins, are believed to be responsible for the anti-depression and calming effect of exercise. Endorphins also may help account for the fact that hunger seems to be diminished for two to three hours

THE DEPRESSED-SLUGGISH-HUNGRY SYNDROME

I vividly remember the fall when I gained twenty pounds. I was depressed. I drank too much red wine with too much dinner every night, and spent a lot of time after my son went to bed lying on the couch eating my way through the big bags of mini candy bars I'd bought for Halloween.
— *Jill*

◆ ◆ ◆

Nearly every woman I know has sunk into this spiral at some time in her life. She feels unhappy and lethargic; she turns to food for comfort and for energy. So she gains weight—and then she feels even worse.

Each of these problems could be addressed individually. She could see a therapist for the depression, lethargy, and low self-esteem; improved nutrition could help her lose weight. But the most effective way to break out of this syndrome is with physical activity. Exercise lifts depression, combats lethargy, and makes weight loss easier. Strengthening exercise is especially helpful, because a woman sees significant changes in just a few weeks.

following vigorous exercise. Another contributor could be the slight elevation in body temperature with exercise, similar to the appetite-depressing effects of fever. Though more research is needed to settle the matter, many women have told me that taking a brisk walk helps them tame between-meal hunger—and this is one appetite suppressant I don't hesitate to recommend.

SIGNALS FROM OUR FAT CELLS

You may have heard of the fat cell theory of overweight—the idea that people reach adulthood with a certain number of fat cells, and that these cells demand to be refilled if they become depleted. There's some truth to this. Our fat cells produce a protein called **leptin** that plays an important role in appetite regulation.

When leptin reaches the hypothalamus, it triggers a receptor that puts the brakes on production of a neurotransmitter called **neuropeptide Y** (NPY). NPY is not only the brain's most potent appetite stimulant, but also a powerful metabolic suppressant. If we lose a little fat, we produce a little less leptin and have a corresponding increase in NPY. In other words, if you eat less on one day, you feel hungrier the next day and eat more.

Many scientists believe that this interaction between leptin and NPY may be responsible for the **set point** for weight—a weight that our body seems to return to, no matter how hard we try to lose. I prefer to use the term **settling point**, because there's evidence that this point is subject to change. One mechanism seems to be physical activity. We know that physical activity creates biochemical changes in the brain—that's why exercise relieves anxiety and depression. Some of these changes appear to affect NPY, which may explain the appetite-suppressing effects of physical activity. Though this hasn't yet been confirmed by research, I suspect we'll eventually have solid evidence that increasing physical activity can actually reset your "normal" weight.

Is Leptin the Answer?

About forty years ago, scientists conducted an experiment in which they surgically connected the blood systems of pairs of mice, one normal and one, called the OB/OB mouse, that had been genetically altered to be overweight. OB/OB mice usually spend their days eating and sleeping; they gain weight rapidly and develop a characteristic round shape. But when these roly-poly mice were connected to normal mice, they suddenly changed their ways: their metabolic rate increased; they ate less, became much more active, and lost weight. Obviously there was something magical in the blood of the normal mice.

In 1994 Jeffrey Friedman, Ph.D., and his colleagues at Rockefeller University finally identified the remarkable substance: leptin. Given leptin, bred-to-be-fat OB/OB mice become slim. Excited by such promising results, a drug company paid $20 million for the commercial rights to leptin. Human studies are under way to see if administering leptin, or making the hypothalamus more sensitive to it, could prevent the surge in NPY that produces raging appetite and sluggish metabolism.

Though this is a very promising area of research, remember that the body has other independent mechanisms that regulate appetite and metabolism. Defects in these systems may account for overweight in some people. If leptin turns out to be the answer, individuals who benefit from leptin treatment probably will have to continue taking it, much as diabetics require insulin.

THE THREE WEIGHT-LOSS STRATEGIES THAT REALLY WORK

If you've ever tried to lose weight, you know it isn't easy. A recent Harris poll reported that women dieters had attempted to lose weight an average of fourteen times! According to a survey by *Prevention* magazine, 70 percent of women who go on a diet hit a plateau before they reach their goal. Discouraged, nearly all of them give up and return to their previous eating habits.

Yes, weight loss is difficult—as I've just explained, your metabolic system and appetite seem determined to thwart your efforts. But we're learning that with the right approach, you can break through. New findings on the benefits of strength training are enormously encouraging. Another source of helpful new insights is the National Weight Control Registry, an exciting project at the University of Pittsburgh. Investigators have located hundreds of men and women who have been able to take off significant amounts of weight and keep it off. They've just published the first in what I hope will be a series of reports about their volunteers—629 women and 155 men who have lost an average of sixty-six pounds, and have maintained at least thirty pounds of that loss for an average of five and a half years.

The latest research indicates that three strategies are the key to successful long-term weight loss:

#1: BUILD LEAN TISSUE BY STRENGTH TRAINING

The more muscle you have, the more calories you burn. This important change comes partly from a revved-up metabolism and partly from increased physical activity—an automatic consequence of greater strength. Strengthening exercise also protects your muscle and bone, so you don't lose precious lean tissue along with fat.

#2: GET MOVING!

Experts now agree that most people are overweight not because they eat too much but because they exercise too little. Vigorous aerobic exercise—the kind that makes you breathe harder—is just part of what's needed. Even more important is increasing your activity throughout the day. The more energetically you move, the more calories you will burn. The crucial importance of exercise for maintaining weight loss is underscored by the experience of the successful dieters in the National Weight Control Registry: an astonishing 89 percent of them were physically active.

#3: FLY JUST BELOW YOUR BODY'S HUNGER RADAR

Cutting calories is usually necessary. However, most women can lose weight successfully on a wholesome, well-balanced diet that supplies 1600 to 2000 calories per day—provided they're physically active. If you try to speed weight loss by reducing food intake more drastically, you might lose a few extra pounds for a couple of weeks. But restrictive, quick-loss diets are doomed by catastrophic metabolic drops. In the long run, you'll lose more weight—and keep it off more easily—if you eat more. A generous food plan is not only more enjoyable and more satisfying, it also provides more nutrients and thereby reduces hunger and cravings.

The *Strong Women Stay Slim* program is designed to help you do all this. Perhaps the best part of the program is that you don't have to compromise your health to take advantage of these weight-loss strategies. Indeed, as you'll see in Chapters 3 and 4, the same changes that will make you slim will have many other wonderful benefits.

▼   ▼   ▼   ▼   ▼   ▼

3

HOW EXERCISE
TRANSFORMS YOUR BODY

*I knew exercise was really important, but I was having a lot of
trouble getting into it. I had a project at work that kept me sedentary; I had two little children at home—and I wasn't happy with
myself. When I started strength training, everything became easier. After my legs got stronger, I began using a stationary bike.
Then I added sit-ups. In a couple of months I lost ten pounds.*
     — Martha

◆   ◆   ◆

Sometimes, after I've given a lecture that describes the remarkable benefits of physical activity, a woman will come up to me and say:

I'll start exercising after I lose weight.

If I ask her why she doesn't want to begin right away, she says:

*What's the point in trying to get fit if I'm overweight? And besides,
there's no way I'm going to a gym, riding my bike, or getting into
a bathing suit when I look like this.*

Ironically, the heavier a woman is, the more she will benefit from exercise. As I explained in Chapter 2, physical activity is the key to lasting weight loss. But that's not all. Exercise breaks through the sluggishness and depression that keep a woman stuck in unhealthy patterns she desperately wants to change. Getting active—even before she loses weight—gives her a new sparkle that makes her look and feel more attractive. The change goes deeper. Scientists now suspect that many of the medical problems blamed on overweight are actually caused in large part by inactivity.

AN EPIDEMIC OF WEAKNESS

Behind the epidemic of overweight in the United States is another epidemic that has gotten very little attention: the weakening of American women. A recent national study of 10,000 women age 40 to 55 found that more than a quarter of them were so weak that they had difficulty with everyday activities—climbing a flight of stairs, carrying groceries, or walking around the block. The heavier the woman, the more likely she was to experience disabling weakness.

What's happening to our strength? I've already explained that many women lose muscle when they diet. An inactive lifestyle also plays a role—"Use it or lose it" definitely applies to muscles. Even more pervasive is the shift in body composition that begins in midlife. Starting around age 40, we typically lose muscle mass at the rate of about a third of a pound a year, and we gain that much body fat or more. If nothing is done to prevent it, by age 80 we'll have only a third of the muscle we had at age 40. This change, called *sarcopenia* (from the Greek "sarco" for muscle or flesh and "penia" for loss) is one of the chief reasons for frailty and loss of vitality later in life.

The spiral of weakness and inactivity—which leads to further muscle loss and weakness—also explains why so many women put on weight as they get older. With less muscle they burn fewer calories, so it becomes easier and easier to gain. But when women start strength training, changes move in the other direction.

STARTING OFF STRONG

I hated the idea of exercise, but strength training sounded tolerable: I wouldn't have to wear special clothes, get down on the floor, move rapidly, or sweat. So I started lifting weights, and—surprise!—I was good at it. This got me interested in trying other exercise for the first time in my life.
— Sarah

◆ ◆ ◆

Strengthening exercise prepares your body for a more active lifestyle. A big part is that you're getting stronger, but there's more: strength training also improves your balance and flexibility, reducing your risk of injury.

GAINS IN STRENGTH, NOT BULK

Strength training enlarges muscle cells, enabling them to exert more force. When women hear this, they often worry that strength training will give them a bulky "Ms. Olympia" look. However, that doesn't happen on the *Strong Women Stay Slim* program. Female body builders follow a very different regimen. They lift much heavier weights and have lengthier workouts; some also take steroids and follow rigorous diets. The women in my studies don't go to these extremes. They become a lot stronger, but they usually wind up *smaller*, not larger. For example, in my *JAMA* osteoporosis study, volunteers gained only about three pounds of muscle, but that was enough to make an enormous difference in their strength. At the same time, they lost three pounds of fat. Since a pound of fat takes up more room than a pound of muscle, they became trimmer, not bulkier.

Increased strength isn't just a matter of bigger muscles. Two other changes are also important:

- ◆ **Nerve reactivation**—Muscles move when signals flash
  from the brain via nerves, telling muscle fibers to contract.
  Strength is lost not only because muscles shrink if they're
  inactive, but also because muscle-stimulating nerves
  become dormant. Strength training reactivates these
  nerves almost immediately, bringing more muscle cells

into play. That's why you'll see big results quickly, without much change in muscle size.

◆ **Enzyme enhancements**—As strength training stimulates your muscles, certain beneficial enzymes increase, improving your body's ability to process oxygen and fuel. This change also contributes to strength.

◆ ◆ ◆

I have been strength training for about ten weeks, and it amazes me how quickly my body has responded. I'd been walking on a treadmill for thirty minutes, three times a week, for approximately a year. I had been stuck at the same speed for several months, not due to cardiovascular difficulty but because my legs would get too fatigued. Since starting strength training, I have increased my speed twice and am not having any problems with my legs. I'm thrilled!
— Denise

◆ ◆ ◆

BETTER BALANCE

Our balancing ability starts to decline in midlife. This change happens so slowly that most of us don't notice it until we're in our seventies. Strength training helps to halt the deterioration and turn it around. In my *JAMA* osteoporosis study, the women who didn't exercise scored 8.5 percent lower on a balance test after just one year. In contrast, the volunteers who strength trained showed a dramatic improvement: their balance test scores increased by 14 percent.

We know that older women are very much aware of impaired balance, and many curtail their physical activity to avoid falling. Younger women also may become less active in response to subtle changes in their balance. Regardless of your age, improved balance will certainly reduce your risk of falls and injury—and may also boost your physical self-confidence.

IMPROVED FLEXIBILITY

When your joints are flexible, sports and other physical activities become much easier. Although flexibility has not been the main focus of my research, many of my volunteers are delighted to find that their shoulders, knees, and ankles become much more flexible as a result of strength training.

◆ ◆ ◆

Last year, if I sat on the floor with my legs straight in front of me and I bent forward, I could barely reach two inches beyond my knees. Now, after eight months of strength training, I can stretch fourteen inches farther and almost touch my toes.
—Judith

◆ ◆ ◆

EXERCISE EXTENDS AND IMPROVES YOUR LIFE

If doctors could prescribe exercise in pill form, it would be the single most widely prescribed drug in the world.
—Robert Butler, M.D., founding director of the
National Institute on Aging

◆ ◆ ◆

Dr. Butler is one of my favorite mentors, and this is my favorite quote about exercise. Strength training has powerful health benefits. You gain even more because your new strength encourages you to become more active.

When I was a graduate student in the early 1980s, we were just beginning to realize that physical activity could reduce the risk of cardiovascular disease. Back then we also knew that being active was important for weight control. It's been exciting to watch the list of benefits expand every year. Accumulated evidence was so extensive by 1996 that the Surgeon General of the United States, in collaboration with the Centers for Disease Control and Prevention, issued a special report on physical activity that concluded:

Moderate exercise is just as essential to a healthy life as good nutrition, seat belts, and avoiding cigarettes.

People who exercise regularly not only live longer, they live *better*. They're healthier and have fewer disabilities; they're happier and more productive—and they look better too. What's more, all these gains come with few, if any, negative consequences.

PERFECT PARTNERS

Strengthening exercise is enormously valuable—but it doesn't train your heart and lungs. For that you need **aerobic exercise**. An aerobic activity is one that causes your heart to beat faster and your breathing rate to increase. This happens during the exercise because your muscles are working and calling for more fuel and oxygen.

Aerobic exercise is the perfect complement to strength training, especially if you want to lose weight. Here's what it adds:

- Burns calories, which contributes to weight loss and loss of fat generally.

- Helps burn fat in your abdominal area.

- Aids in toning your muscles.

- Tames your appetite, bringing it in line with your energy expenditure.

- Provides an emotional lift.

- Improves the health of your cardiovascular system and lungs.

BEING FIT HELPS EVEN IF YOU'RE OVERWEIGHT

Much of what we know about the relationship between lifestyle and health comes from ambitious research projects that follow thousands of people over many years. Steven Blair, P.E.D., and his colleagues at the Cooper Institute for Aerobics Research in Dallas, Texas, have done the largest such study focusing on exercise. Since 1970 they've recruited over 25,000 men and more than 7,000 women age 20 to 88, all of whom agreed to be followed for seven to eight

THE #1 QUESTION WOMEN ASK ABOUT EXERCISE

I recently gave a talk about strength training at a retirement community, and afterward I asked if anyone had questions. An attractive elderly woman immediately raised her hand. "I'm 88 years old," she said. "What can I do to firm up my abs?" I hear this question all the time, from teenagers on up.

Here's how strength training and aerobic exercise deliver a one-two punch to firm and flatten your abdominal area:

◆ Strengthening exercise tones the muscles in your abdomen and back. It's easy to understand why the abdominal muscles are important, but how do the back muscles affect your appearance in front? Strong back muscles contribute to good posture, which makes your abdomen look flatter. Women who have poor posture look thicker around the middle.

◆ Aerobic exercise not only burns calories, but also specifically targets the layer of fat in the abdominal area, which is bad for health as well as appearance. In addition, certain aerobic activities—including walking, cycling, stair climbing, and cross-country skiing—help firm the abdominal and back muscles.

years. These volunteers underwent extensive physical examinations—including a treadmill test to assess fitness—and provided detailed personal information. The researchers know the volunteers' height and weight, their blood pressure and cholesterol profiles, their smoking habits, and their medical histories.

In 1996 Dr. Blair and his associates wrote a fascinating report focused on those participants—601 men and 89 women—who died during their follow-up period. What was the biggest difference between the volunteers who died and the ones who survived? Not fat, but fitness. When other risk factors were held constant, those in the lowest fitness category had double the mortality rate of those whose fitness was medium or high. The findings were startling: fitness trumped all other risk factors, including overweight, diabetes, elevated blood pressure, and high cholesterol. Only smoking came close.

People who were fat and fit had the same mortality risk as people who were lean and fit—and *much lower* mortality rates than those who were lean but unfit. Other research has confirmed these findings: **being fit helps you live longer—no matter how much you weigh.**

EXERCISE TURNS BACK THE CLOCK

My mother lives in an assisted-living facility. When I visit her I see women in their eighties and nineties, who never were encouraged to do anything physical—and now their lives are so impaired by their disabilities. That's prompted me to take active steps.
—Judith

♦   ♦   ♦

As you can see, physical activity has extraordinary rejuvenating effects. I'm not just talking about feeling more youthful, though of course that's one result. Exercise actually alters the body in ways that reverse or compensate for age-related declines.

After a year of strength training, the postmenopausal women in my *JAMA* study showed remarkable changes. Without taking drugs, they regained bone instead of losing it as women normally do at that age. They became stronger—in most cases stronger than they'd ever been in their lives. Their balance and flexibility improved. Because movement was so much easier, they spontaneously became more physically active. When we took stock of all these changes, we realized that *after just one year of strength training their bodies had become fifteen to twenty years more youthful.*

Aerobic exercise revitalizes your cardiovascular system. Typically we lose cardiovascular fitness as we get older, especially if we're not active. One reason is that after age 40, our hearts gradually lose the ability to beat rapidly, so our maximum heart rate begins to decline. This change occurs even in those who remain physically fit, which helps explain why the performance of top athletes usually peaks when they're in their twenties and thirties. But few of us challenge our hearts to perform anywhere near their maximum. Far more significant for most women are the changes that result from inactivity—but these can be largely reversed by aerobic exercise. A study I did in the mid-1980s found that physically active women age 50 to 70 had the same level of cardiovascular fitness as sedentary women half their age.

EXERCISE FIGHTS DISEASE AND DISABILITY

Physical activity makes a major contribution to health simply by helping women lose weight and keep it off. But the benefits go further. In addition, physical activity reduces the risk for many diseases; it may also counter symptoms if you already have a medical condition. Here's an up-to-the-minute summary—but I can promise that as additional research is completed, there will be even more.

Cardiovascular Disease

Cardiovascular disease—heart disease and stroke—is the number-one killer of both women and men. Overweight people have triple the normal risk. The best way to combat the danger is by a combination of weight loss, improved diet, and physical activity. But exercise is beneficial all by itself: it reduces blood pressure, decreases the level of harmful cholesterol in the blood, and improves the condition of blood vessels. These changes greatly reduce the risk of heart attacks and stroke.

Aerobic exercise conditions your cardiovascular system in three ways:

- ◆ Increases the amount of blood you can pump with each heartbeat, which compensates for age-related limitations.

- ◆ Improves circulation by making your blood vessels healthier.

- ◆ Increases production of enzymes responsible for oxygen metabolism, allowing you to use oxygen more effectively.

What does this mean in real life? When your cardiovascular fitness improves, you have more energy; you don't find yourself gasping for breath if you have to move quickly. Activities that stopped being enjoyable because they were such a struggle become fun again.

Diabetes

An estimated 15 million Americans have diabetes, and about half of them don't even know it. The disease, which interferes with sugar metabolism, kills more than 150,000 people a year and is one of the largest contributors to heart disease. Overweight is strongly associated with adult-onset diabetes, by far the more prevalent form. By countering overweight, exercise works indirectly to reduce the risk of diabetes. In addition, physical activity contributes to metabolic changes that allow the body to process sugar more efficiently.

Cancer

Women are often surprised to hear that exercise can actually decrease their cancer risk, but studies of large groups of people show there really is a connection—especially with breast and colon cancer. What's the link? In the case of breast cancer, the most likely explanation has to do with hormones. We make estrogens in our body fat, so the more fat we have, the more estrogen exposure we get. The greater our estrogen exposure, the higher our breast cancer risk. Exercise probably protects against colon cancer by helping to speed wastes through the digestive tract. This gives carcinogens less time to act on the lining of the colon.

Arthritis and Joint Problems

About 20 million Americans suffer from one or more forms of arthritis, diseases of the joints. Excess weight is often a contributing factor, especially in osteoarthritis: the joints of the ankles, knees, and hips don't get any larger if you gain weight, but they have to work a lot harder. People who suffer from arthritis often lose muscle and become weaker, not only because their mobility is impaired but also because of the medications they take. In the past, people with arthritis were advised not to exercise, for fear of causing pain and further damage to the joints. However, several important new studies have shown that both strength training and aerobic exercise not only are safe but also provide pain relief, and improve mobility and strength.

Osteoporosis

This devastating condition, in which bones become dangerously fragile, affects about 25 million Americans, mostly women over age 50. But preventive measures should begin decades earlier. The more bone mass a woman can accumulate before menopause, the larger her reserves later in life.

For someone with osteoporosis, an accidental fall can mean broken bones, disability, and even death. Indeed, more women die each year from hip fractures related to osteoporosis than from breast cancer, uterine cancer, and ovarian cancer combined! My *JAMA* study showed that strength training just two times a week dramatically cuts the risk of osteoporosis by restoring bone, building strength, and improving balance, thereby reducing the risk of falls. Other research has demonstrated that weight-bearing aerobic activities, such as calisthenics and walking, are also beneficial. We don't yet have long-term data on osteoporosis risk in women who do both strength training *and* aerobic exercise. But my guess is that they will enjoy the greatest protection of all.

ACTIVE WOMEN ARE HAPPIER

I'm a secretary, and I sit in front of a computer all day. I've finally started to understand my body when it tells me I need to exercise. Maybe I'm a little depressed and I know that if I take a walk, I'll feel better. Or I get stiff and crabby at the same time, and I make the connection—my body is telling me to do something.
　　—Therese

◆　◆　◆

My favorite way to unwind after a hectic week is to go into the woods behind our house and take a long walk. No matter how much tension has built up, after a brisk walk I feel peaceful and relaxed. Research suggests that many women have the same response to exercise. There's evidence that physical activity enhances mood, improves coping skills, and boosts self-esteem and self-confidence. Active people are only half as likely as their sedentary counterparts to suffer from the bouts of anxiety and depression that plague nearly three out of every ten Americans.

All this is especially good news for a woman who finds herself turning to food in response to stress or unhappiness—and then feeling worse because she gains weight. Exercise gives her a way to get unstuck.

BEING ACTIVE MAKES WOMEN FEEL BETTER ABOUT THEMSELVES

Self-esteem and self-confidence are the fundamentals of mental health. Do you like yourself? Do you believe you can accomplish what you want to do? For many overweight women, the answer is "No." For starters, problems with self-esteem and self-confidence are more common in women than in men. Excess weight adds to the emotional burden. Looking back on how she felt before she started strength training, Martha told me:

> *I avoided going to social events because I wasn't pleased with what I looked like and my clothes didn't fit. I didn't feel good about myself. I wasn't proud of myself. I had a problem I wasn't dealing with, so I felt out of control.*

Exercise turns these feelings around almost immediately. When women lose weight as well, the transformation is almost magical. Martha says:

> *I take such pleasure in my progress—more pleasure and more comfort than I used to find in food. I feel in control and I'm happier about everything.*

FITNESS FIGHTS DEPRESSION

Some people get such a delightful boost from vigorous exercise that they describe themselves as feeling high. Actually, they may not be wrong. Scientists speculate that aerobic exercise improves mood by stimulating production of endorphins, chemicals in the brain that have effects similar to opiates. Indeed, the word "endorphin" comes from the same root as "morphine."

We've known for years about the depression-fighting benefits of aerobic exercise. Now we're learning that strength training is equally helpful. A study done in our laboratory by Nalin Singh, M.D., and colleagues looked at thirty-two men and women who suffered from chronic depression. Half the volunteers did strength training; the others simply received health education. Twelve weeks later, fourteen out of the sixteen members of the strength training group felt so much better that they no longer met the clinical criteria for depression, but only six members of the education-only group enjoyed similar relief. This impressive success rate is comparable to that produced by highly effective anti-depressants.

Physical Activity Reduces Anxiety and Stress

Many women tell me—and research confirms—that one of the best benefits of exercise is that their stress levels drop. They feel calmer and more relaxed in general. Also, they now turn to exercise rather than to food when they face stress-provoking situations.

♦　♦　♦

I go to a massage therapist because of tension in my neck and right shoulder. After I started strength training, she noticed that my whole upper body seemed more opened up. My shoulders were held back naturally, and I didn't have that round-shouldered look.
　—Jane

♦　♦　♦

Exercise Is Better Than a Sleeping Pill

Active people have more energy during the day, and they sleep better at night. In scientific studies, many measures of sleep quality show improvements: people who get regular exercise fall asleep more quickly, sleep more deeply, awaken less often in the middle of the night, and sleep longer. These benefits are comparable to those of medication, but with none of the side effects.

Now that researchers are exploring the effects of strength training, we're finding similar results. In Dr. Singh's study of depression, ten people in the strength-training group, and seven in the health-education group, reported sleep problems when they joined the project. After twelve weeks, six of the ten strength-training volunteers reported that they no longer had difficulty sleeping; in contrast, no one in the health-education group improved.

A LITTLE BIT MAKES A BIG DIFFERENCE

You might assume that adding a little exercise would give you just a little benefit. That's true for those who are already exercising vigorously—doing more doesn't make a big difference for health. But small changes can have major effects for sedentary people. In Dr. Blair's study at the Cooper Institute for Aerobics Research, which I described earlier in this chapter, the most dramatic drop in mortality came when people changed from being totally sedentary to moderately active. **The more inactive you are now, the more you will benefit from exercise.**

Strength training delivers significant improvements with just two or three thirty-minute sessions per week. For aerobic exercise, three to five thirty-minute workouts per week suffice. You don't even have to engage in planned exercise to benefit. Simply being more active in everyday life—walking more, climbing more stairs, spending more time on active hobbies like gardening and golf—improves health and reduces mortality.

The *Strong Women Stay Slim* program will gently ease you into a more active lifestyle. Strength training and aerobic exercise will help you lose weight and keep it off. But the beauty of exercise is that it does so much more. Because you're reducing the risk for many chronic diseases and disabilities, you're increasing the odds that you'll live a long and healthy life. The benefits begin immediately, even before you shed a pound. You'll have a surge of energy and a tremendous sense of pride in what you're accomplishing.

EATING FOR HEALTH AND PLEASURE

I need a lot of flexibility. This plan allowed me to eat well, to make choices, and to give myself a treat. If I really wanted butter on my bread, I could have it. If I baked cookies with the kids, I could eat one. I could have a drink before dinner. It made all the difference to me that I had the leeway and the freedom.
— *Nancy*

◆　◆　◆

On Sunday mornings I serve waffles for breakfast, a wonderful tradition from my husband's family. Guests who join us for the first time often are surprised to see me—a nutritionist—piling my plate with waffles and fruit, and topping the stack with sour cream and maple syrup. But there's nothing wrong with this meal. It's a perfectly reasonable part of the well-rounded diet and active lifestyle that keep me and my family healthy and slender. Even with this indulgence, our weekly consumption of fats and sweets is within guidelines for good nutrition. During the rest of the day we more than compensate for the extra calories with vigorous physical activity.

The best way to lose weight is through a combination of exercise and a wholesome food plan that lets you take pleasure in eating again. Good nutrition becomes particularly important when you're trying to lose weight. Not only do you need to select the right foods for weight loss, you also want to be sure they deliver the essentials you need. Scientists now know a great deal about the optimal diet for health and longevity. But only you can determine how to adapt this information to your life and your preferences—and that's a key part of staying slim. Yes, you can lose weight on a diet you don't like. But how will you maintain the loss? A food plan you enjoy is one you will follow for a lifetime.

EATING SHOULD BE A PLEASURE

When I sit down for a meal with women friends and relatives, I'm often dismayed to hear comments like these:

I shouldn't be eating this.
I've wrecked the whole week with this meal.

For many women, eating is fraught with guilt and unhappiness. Instead of savoring the delicious food served on special occasions—family gatherings, dinner parties with friends, and holiday celebrations at the office—they worry about losing control and eating too much. A tiny bit of guilt is a superb motivator, but beyond that it's counterproductive. When you feel guilty about food, it's easy to fall into a negative spiral of self-criticism, poor self-image, and even depression—which leads to overeating and more bad feelings. This is one reason that overly restrictive diets seldom work in the long run.

When you need to control the *quantity* of food you eat, it becomes even more important to enjoy the *quality*. The pleasure that you get from eating is a significant part of life. You don't have to turn your back on it; rather, you have to harness this potent motivator. Here are three basic principles for maximizing enjoyment as you lose weight:

◆ EAT TO THE LIMIT

You can't lose weight unless your caloric intake is consistently less than your caloric expenditure. But the gap should be as small as possible while still allowing you to lose. It's not just a matter of minimizing deprivation, though that's a very important goal. The more you eat, the more nutrients your diet can provide, and the healthier and more satisfying it will be. As you may have experienced yourself, women who cut back too much can send their body into starvation mode, thwarting their efforts to lose. Their metabolic rate drops; they become lethargic and therefore burn fewer calories through physical activity; and their appetite screams for food.

◆ INCLUDE YOUR FAVORITE FOODS

I'm not saying you're going to be able to eat any amount of everything you might want. But if you take great pleasure in certain foods, it's important to have them in appropriate quantities so you don't feel deprived.

Lillian sometimes says that the secret of her successful weight loss is peanut butter. She'd been slim all her life, then went through a difficult period in her early fifties and gained twenty pounds. When she finally decided to go on a diet, she wanted quick results. She selected a plan that had worked well for a friend, even though it prohibited peanut butter and other foods she enjoys. She lost the twenty pounds in just three months, but a year later the weight was back. After several more yo-yo cycles she came to me. "I rebound on peanut butter," she said. "I love it, but I know I shouldn't eat it because it's so fattening."

"If you enjoy peanut butter, there's no reason you can't have it," I told her. We worked out nutritious meal plans that incorporated reasonable portions of peanut butter and her other favorites. Six months later, Lillian's excess weight was gone—and she's maintained the loss for three years.

◆ CULTIVATE NEW PREFERENCES

When you're losing weight, it's not enough to restrict calories—it's also important to eat a healthy variety of foods so you get all the nutrients your body needs. An astonishing abundance is available in stores and produce markets today, but we sometimes limit ourselves to what's familiar. Alexandra told me that sweets were her downfall. A few weeks after she started the program, when we discussed her food diary, I congratulated her on cutting back

WHERE DO FOOD CRAVINGS COME FROM?

Cravings sometimes reflect actual physical needs, either for specific nutrients or for food in general. Though we don't yet have solid research on this, many clinical nutritionists have noticed that when their clients begin eating a varied, well-balanced diet and get enough food, their cravings are greatly reduced.

Another source of cravings is emotional. We associate certain foods with comfort or good times, so we may yearn for them when we're under stress. Adding to this effect is the fact that high-carbohydrate foods increase the brain's supply of serotonin, a mood-affecting chemical.

her dessert portions. But I also noted that her fruit consumption was limited to orange juice, raisins, and apples. "I've never liked fruit," she explained. "Besides, it's too much trouble to prepare." I suggested she try one new fruit per week. She agreed to start with ready-to-eat melon chunks from the salad bar at her supermarket.

One year later, Alexandra's tastes had expanded considerably. She recently e-mailed me this update:

> We had friends over the other night, and I served fresh pineapple and cookies. The pineapple was so luscious that I took seconds and ignored the cookies. Afterward, when I realized what I'd done, I was absolutely stunned: I've become one of those people who eats fruit for dessert!

CALORIES ALWAYS COUNT

One way or another, *all* weight reduction diets restrict food energy so that intake is lower than energy expenditure. Some keep track of calories. Others, including the food plan in this book, focus on portions instead, but that's just a simpler way to count calories.

A less obvious way to restrict calories is to limit your food choices. Some "calories don't count" plans limit dieters to just a few specific foods; others rule out entire categories. The secret of their temporary success is that most people get bored with the permitted foods, and they eat less. However, that very same boredom makes the diet all but impossible to follow for a lifetime, so the weight returns.

GOOD NUTRITION FOR WEIGHT LOSS

Any diet that cuts calories enough can produce weight loss. I hope you're looking for a lot more—good nutrition, practicality, flexibility, and enjoyment. These are the considerations I keep in mind when I review research about the best diets for weight control.

The food plan in this book, which I'll detail in Chapter 9, is based on the Food Guide Pyramid. This blueprint for nutritious eating distills decades of research about the relationship between diet and longevity and optimal health—large-scale surveys, as well as meticulous laboratory investigations. Experts have struggled for years to translate all this information into practical advice. Since 1941, the government has issued nutrient-by-nutrient guidelines for a healthy diet: the Recommended Dietary Allowances (RDAs). Most Americans became familiar with the RDAs from food labels. But many people were intimidated by the long lists of vitamins and minerals; they had dif-

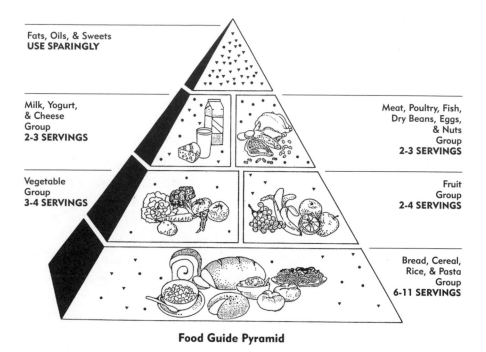

Food Guide Pyramid

ficulty translating milligrams into menus for daily meals. So in 1980 the U.S. Department of Agriculture and the Department of Health and Human Services assembled a group of the nation's leading experts—doctors, nutritionists, scientists, and communications specialists—to come up with a simpler approach. The panel suggested new guidelines that focused on foods and portions, rather than on nutrients, like the RDAs. The eventual result was the Food Guide Pyramid.

In Chapter 9 I'll show you how to translate these guidelines into daily menus that give you all the nutrients you need. And there's plenty of room for adjustments to allow for your preferences.

THE ESSENTIAL INGREDIENTS

The *Strong Women Stay Slim* food plan optimizes the Food Guide Pyramid for weight loss, while retaining as much flexibility as possible. While you're losing weight you'll be well nourished. Afterward, you can use the same structure for a lifetime of healthy eating. Here are the basic components this plan provides:

CARBOHYDRATES

Many women are confused about carbohydrates—and no wonder. Some experts recommend that you eat them in abundance when you're dieting, while others warn that you must carefully limit them to lose weight. Women often ask me questions about high-carbohydrate foods:

Will pasta make me fat?
Should I be eating potatoes?
Is it bad to have bread?

Most nutritionists—including me—consider carbohydrates the staff of life. They're the body's chief source of fuel, providing most of the energy

THE GLYCEMIC INDEX

The glycemic index is a measure of how rapidly the carbohydrates in a food are broken down and turned into sugar in the blood. You may have heard about weight-loss approaches that feature a blanket recommendation against foods that have a high glycemic index. There's no scientific basis for avoiding all such foods—a list that would include carrots, bananas, potatoes, pasta, and whole-grain bread. On the contrary, there's plenty of evidence to suggest that these items are good for you. They supply valuable nutrients, and scientific surveys show that people who consume a diet high in these complex carbohydrates enjoy above-average health. However, certain high-glycemic foods, like sugary candy, provide nothing but calories. It's also true that a diet with a large amount of high-glycemic foods *plus* a low fiber intake can put you at risk for heart disease and diabetes. And, of course, any food can cause weight gain if consumed in excess.

we need for exercise and everything else we do. Carbohydrates also play an important role in satisfying our appetite: as they're converted into sugar and enter the bloodstream, they signal to the hypothalamus that we've eaten. When you follow the food plan in this book, about 55 to 60 percent of the calories you consume will be from carbohydrates.

There are two kinds of carbohydrates in food: sugars and starches. On their own, sugars add only flavor and calories to our diet—that's why the Food Guide Pyramid recommends that they be eaten sparingly. This is just as true for "natural" or "unrefined" forms like honey or maple syrup as it is for cane sugar. But you can more freely indulge your sweet tooth with the sugars in fruit because they come with valuable extras. For instance, the sugar in an orange is accompanied by impressive amounts of fiber, vitamin C, folate, potassium, and other valuable nutrients.

Starches—better known these days as "complex carbohydrates"—are found in grains, legumes (peas, beans), potatoes, and other vegetables. Your body has to work harder to digest starch than sugar; this is especially true when the starch is in unrefined grains, because those also contain fiber. That's an advantage when you're trying to lose weight: the slower a food is digested, the longer your appetite feels satisfied. Furthermore, whole grains provide important trace minerals that aren't found in many other foods.

PROTEIN

Protein is the body's chief building material—our muscles, bones, cartilage, skin, hair, and blood are made in part from protein. When you follow the food plan in this book, 15 to 20 percent of your caloric intake is from protein.

We use many different kinds of protein, but all are combinations of the same twenty amino acids. Our body manufactures eleven of these acids, but the other nine—the essential amino acids—must be obtained from food. It's easy to get enough if you eat animal products. For weight loss, low-fat versions are best.

Certain plant foods contain protein too, but these proteins lack one or more of the nine essential amino acids. Fortunately for vegetarians, different plants contain different amino acids. Well-chosen combinations—including traditional favorites such as rice and beans or corn and beans—can provide a complete set.

The question I'm most frequently asked about protein is this:

If protein helps build muscle, can extra protein give me added muscle and strength?

No—there's no scientific evidence that it can. One of my colleagues, Wayne Campbell, Ph.D., investigated this question in a careful study that was published in the *American Journal of Clinical Nutrition* in 1994. Twelve men and women volunteered to spend twelve weeks living in our metabolic unit at Tufts, so that everything they ate and everything they excreted could be measured. Half of them consumed the recommended amount of protein, and half were given a diet with double that amount. The volunteers also did vigorous strength training to build muscles. At the end of twelve weeks, there was no difference between the two groups in muscle tissue and strength. Other studies have since corroborated this finding.

THE PROBLEM WITH HIGH-PROTEIN/LOW-CARBOHYDRATE DIETS

If you cut carbohydrates drastically and add a corresponding amount of protein, your body is forced to turn to an inferior fuel source: fat metabolites called ketones. Because ketones are toxic, your kidneys go into overdrive to flush them out of your system. In the process, you drain water from your tissues. Since a pint of water weighs about a pound, you can lose an impressive amount of weight very quickly on a high-protein/low-carbohydrate diet. And you may drop a few additional pounds because you're eating less.

There's good news at the scale, perhaps, but bad news for your body. You've lost mainly water—along with calcium from your bones and protein from your muscles—but not as much fat as you think. Moreover, your kidneys are under stress; you may become dehydrated, which puts an extra strain on your heart. Many women become weak after a week or more on a ketogenic diet. Their heart may race or they may become dizzy from minor exertion; they often develop bad breath and other problems. Few people can—or should—stay on this kind of diet in the long run. The weight usually returns quickly as the body's water supply is restored.

Fat

If you're trying to lose weight you may think of fat as the enemy, but that's not quite fair. We all need fat in our diet. Fat supplies two essential nutrients—linoleic acid and linolenic acid —that are necessary for formation of prostaglandins, which are hormone-like compounds that help control reproduction, blood pressure, and other important functions. Fat is also important for appetite control. Because it's broken down more slowly than carbohydrate and protein, it keeps you feeling full longer after a meal. Fat also carries flavor and improves texture, making many foods more enjoyable. On this food plan, about 25 percent of your daily caloric intake is from fat.

Getting enough dietary fat is easy because so many foods contain fat. There's fat in oils and butter, obviously, and also in most sources of protein and in dairy foods; grains and legumes also contain small amounts.

Fat becomes a problem when we eat too much of it. Unfortunately, that's easy to do. Fat is more calorie-dense than protein or carbohydrate—9 calories per gram compared to 4. That's why a scoop of high-fat ice cream might have twice as many calories as the same size scoop of low-fat frozen yo-

NON-FAT DOESN'T MEAN NON-FATTENING!

Food manufacturers have done a terrific job of cutting back on excess fat in processed foods. For instance, low-fat and non-fat dairy products allow us to get all the nutritional benefits of milk, yogurt, and cheese, without excessive fat. But you can't assume that all no-fat foods are healthy, or that they're low in calories.

Like many nutritionists, I've been concerned by the proliferation of snacks and desserts that are "non-fat," but high-sugar and high-calorie. Some women consume these products freely, then wonder why they don't lose weight. But very often the non-fat version has just about the same number of calories as the regular version—and sometimes even more.

gurt. Excess food does more damage when it's high in fat. That's because your body can convert *dietary* fat into *stored* fat with very little metabolic effort. Turning 100 extra carbohydrate calories into body fat "costs" 23 calories, so only 77 calories actually get stored. But if the excess 100 calories come from fat, the process is far more efficient and requires only 3 calories—which means that 97 calories become body fat.

Dietary fat can be a problem even for people who aren't overweight, because it affects blood chemistry and can lead to heart disease and stroke. Certain kinds of fat are more harmful than others, so it's important to be selective:

♦ **Saturated fats**—the kind that are solid at room temperature, like butter, lard, and palm oil—come from animal and dairy products, plus a few plants. People whose diet is high in saturated fat tend to have higher levels of both LDL and HDL cholesterol, which puts them at increased risk for heart disease.

WHAT ABOUT CHOLESTEROL?

Cholesterol is essential to life—but it's become almost synonymous with "heart disease" because it can clog the arteries, leading to heart attacks and strokes. The liver manufactures cholesterol, and most of us get extra amounts of it from food. All fat of animal origin—including egg yolks, dairy fat, and the fat from meat and poultry—contains cholesterol; there's none in fat that comes from plants, like cocoa butter or peanut oil.

In the bloodstream, cholesterol is piggybacked on proteins called **lipoproteins. Low-density lipoproteins (LDL)** bring cholesterol to the cells, but they also deposit it on the arteries. For that reason, LDL is called "bad cholesterol." In contrast, the job of the **high-density lipoproteins (HDL)**—"good cholesterol"—is to remove cholesterol from the bloodstream. (To remember the difference, think H for healthy and L for ill.)

- **Trans fatty acid** is vegetable oil that's been made solid by a manufacturing process called hydrogenation. (Look for "hydrogenated vegetable oil" on the label.) In the body, trans fatty acids have effects similar to those of saturated fat. That's why, nutritionally speaking, there's not much difference between butter and solid margarine.

- **Monounsaturated fat** is liquid at room temperature, but becomes partly firm if chilled. Many experts believe that you can lower LDL and increase HDL by substituting monounsaturated fat for saturated fat—for example, dipping your bread in olive oil instead of spreading it with butter.

- **Polyunsaturated fat** remains liquid unless you put it in the freezer. The fat in most vegetable oils is polyunsaturated, as is the fat in cold-water fish, whose fat must stay liquid so the fish can move. These fats seem to be heart-friendly. An added benefit of vegetable oils is that many of them contain vitamin E, which I'll discuss later in this chapter.

DIETARY FIBER

Fiber is one of nature's best appetite suppressants: it fills you up, yet it contains no calories. Plus, fiber sweeps waste through your gastrointestinal tract. This not only prevents constipation and related ills, but also lowers your risk of colon cancer because carcinogens have less time to act on the intestinal lining. Fiber even provides benefits to the heart, since it helps remove cholesterol from the small intestines. The food plan in this book, which calls for plenty of fruits and vegetables, provides ample fiber.

There are two types of fiber, both of which are valuable:

- **Soluble fiber** can absorb water, turning into a soft gel. It's found in fruits, legumes, oats, rye, and barley.

- **Insoluble fiber** is the kind that doesn't absorb water. Sources include whole wheat products, bran, and fruit and vegetable skins.

Most Americans don't get enough fiber, but that doesn't mean you should sprinkle bran on your food. In excessive quantities, fiber speeds helpful substances—including essential minerals like calcium, iron, and zinc—out of the body before they can be absorbed. Also, too much fiber can irritate the bowel. However, when fiber is consumed as part of whole foods, it's almost impossible to get too much.

WATER

Water is another important weight-loss aid. Though it contains no calories, it contributes to fullness. Many women have told me that they're satisfied with smaller portions when they sip water along with a meal. But that's just one reason it's important to drink enough when you're trying to take off weight. The body uses water for most of its behind-the-scenes processes, from digesting food to sweating. You probably know that you need extra water when you exercise. It's also very important for maintaining energy throughout the day. Many people who feel lethargic don't realize that the reason isn't always lack of sleep; rather, they may be slightly dehydrated. That's why a glass of cool water can be a surprisingly helpful pick-me-up. The *Strong Women Stay Slim* food plan recommends that you get at least eight glasses of water or other fluids per day.

ALCOHOL

If alcohol were on the Food Guide Pyramid, it would be in the "use sparingly" category because of the calories it contains. In moderate quantities, alcoholic beverages (especially red wine) appear to increase HDL, which makes them heart-friendly. However, excessive alcohol consumption causes many problems, including nutritional deficiencies—not only because alcohol is sometimes substituted for more nutritious food, but also because it damages the liver and interferes with metabolism of many nutrients.

MINERALS AND VITAMINS

When you follow the food plan in this book, you get all the vitamins and minerals you need. These nutrients contain no calories, but they're essential to good health.

Our teeth and bones are made up of minerals—mainly calcium, but also phosphorus, magnesium, and fluoride. Minerals also are involved in many of the chemical reactions that sustain life, including metabolism, muscle contractions, and the transmission of nerve impulses.

Vitamins contribute to the body's biochemical functioning as well. Thanks to improved diet, including vitamin-enriched grains, we rarely encounter the deficiencies that were once a common cause of disability and death. However, as I'll discuss later in this chapter, we're beginning to learn that some vitamins have additional health-promoting potential if consumed in larger amounts than we typically get from food.

SURPRISING BONUSES FROM FOOD

The Food Guide Pyramid recommends a diet with plenty of fruits, vegetables, and whole grains. That's because large comparative studies have found that people who follow such a diet are healthier and live longer. We don't know all the reasons, but it's clear that vitamins and minerals are only part of the explanation. I'm tremendously excited by a discovery that is still unfolding: that plant foods contain *thousands* of health-promoting chemicals, called **phytochemicals** from the Greek word "phyto" for plant. Consider them yet another benefit you'll get from the food plan in this book.

One type of phytochemical of particular interest to women is **isoflavones**, also known as phytoestrogens—plant estrogens. Isoflavones, which are found in soybeans, are similar to the estrogens produced by your body. They may explain why Asian women, who consume far more soy than American women do, have fewer hip fractures and fewer menopausal symptoms—in fact, there's no word for "hot flashes" in some Asian languages. Many American women take hormone replacement therapy (HRT) to counter problems associated with menopause; unfortunately, the advantages of HRT are counterbalanced by a small increase in the risk of breast cancer.

ANTIOXIDANTS

People don't rust, and we don't spoil the way food can, but our cells are similarly damaged by the same chemical process: **oxidation**. This damage is now believed to be partly responsible for cancer and many degenerative conditions associated with aging, from cataracts to wrinkles. Here's how it happens:

During normal chemical reactions in the body, cells produce oxygen compounds. Some of these compounds are unstable because they're missing an electron. These unbalanced molecules—called free radicals—take electrons from other molecules, which then become unbalanced themselves. This chain reaction of molecular change is what breaks down healthy material during oxidation. Free radicals are produced by normal processes, and also by air pollution, cigarette smoke, and other stresses to the body.

Harmful oxidation is kept in check by substances called **antioxidants**. These have the ability to donate an electron without becoming unduly unstable, so they can neutralize a free radical without creating more. The body produces its own antioxidants, but we also need some from the foods we eat. Antioxidant nutrients include vitamin C, vitamin E, and numerous phytochemicals.

But Asian women get similar benefits from soy, *and* they have very low breast cancer rates. Why? Apparently the isoflavones in soybeans are a less potent form of estrogen, so they're less likely to stimulate tumors in breast tissue.

In the table on the next two pages, I summarize just a few of the promising phytochemicals and the magic they appear to work. As you'll see, a wide variety of fruits, vegetables, legumes, herbs, and grains contribute. How can you possibly take advantage of this natural pharmacy when we don't even know its full extent? The best way is to consume a rainbow of plant-based foods.

Phyto-chemical	What It Appears to Do	Best Food Sources
Isoflavones (also known as phyto-estrogens)	Reduce risk of breast and ovarian cancer, and osteoporosis; also relieve hot flashes	Soybeans and dried beans
Flavonoids	Reduce risk of heart disease by decreasing oxidation of LDL cholesterol	Red wine, apples, celery, cranberries, grapes, black and green tea, onions
Lutein and zeaxanthin (found together in foods)	Reduce risk for macular degeneration, the leading cause of blindness in older people	Yellow, orange, and dark green leafy vegetables
Ellagic acid	Protects against carcinogens found in tobacco and environmental pollutants	Grapes, strawberries, raspberries
Allyl sulfides	Reduce cancer risk by helping to neutralize carcinogens; also may interfere with reproduction of tumor cells	Garlic, onions, leeks, chives

PHYTO-CHEMICAL	WHAT IT APPEARS TO DO	BEST FOOD SOURCES
Terpenes	Block development of cancer tumors (tamoxifen and taxol, which are used to treat breast cancer, are both terpenes)	Citrus fruits
Isothiocyanates	Trigger the formation of enzymes that could prevent carcinogens from damaging DNA	Cruciferous vegetables like broccoli, cabbage, and cauliflower
Indoles	Reduce the risk of breast cancer by helping the body convert a potentially harmful form of estrogen into a harmless form	Cruciferous vegetables like broccoli, cabbage, and cauliflower
Saponins	Prevent cancer cells from multiplying	Soybeans and other dried beans, cherries
Lycopene	Decreases risk for prostate cancer, probably by reducing DNA damage from oxidation of cells. May decrease other cancers for women	Tomatoes (for lycopene to be absorbed, it must be consumed with some fat)

DO WE NEED SUPPLEMENTS?

As a nutritionist, I'm asked about supplements all the time, not only in the office and at lectures, but also by family and friends. The question isn't easy to answer, because it takes years of research to prove that a supplement provides real benefits and has no harmful side effects. Until recently I never thought about taking supplements myself or recommending them to others, except during pregnancy. Instead I'd suggest consuming a wide variety of wholesome foods. After all, pills can't possibly replace a well-rounded diet because there are so many unknown beneficial components of food. However, I'm beginning to reconsider. New research suggests that even people who choose their foods carefully might benefit from additional amounts of certain nutrients.

CALCIUM

We all know that our bones are made from calcium, and that a high-calcium diet helps keep them strong. But not everyone realizes that calcium is also an essential part of the body's biochemistry: it's needed for contraction of muscles (including the heart), for blood clotting, and for nerve conduction. Indeed, calcium is so important that if we don't get enough in our diet, our body is forced to draw it from our bones.

Just how much is enough for optimal bone health? This is the subject of some controversy, but I believe that current evidence supports the new dietary calcium RDAs issued in 1997 by the National Academy of Sciences: 1000 milligrams daily for women age 18 to 50; 1200 milligrams for women over 50. If you decide to take a calcium supplement, choose a dose that reflects what you're already consuming in your diet. If you follow the food plan in this book, which includes two or three servings of dairy foods, your daily calcium intake will be around 700 to 800 milligrams per day; a sufficient supplement would be 300 milligrams if you're 50 or under, or 500 milligrams if you're older.

VITAMIN D

Calcium gets all the attention, but vitamin D is equally important: without this vitamin your body can't effectively use the calcium you consume. We get vitamin D from food and from the sun, which stimulates our skin cells to manufacture it. All you need is ten minutes of full sunlight to get your daily supply. However, that's usually not possible in the winter, especially if you live in a northern state or province. The best food sources are fortified milk and fortified cereal, but many women don't get enough. If you're among them, I suggest a supplement that supplies 400 to 700 international units (IU) (but don't go above 1000 IU, because vitamin D is toxic at high levels).

A BONE-FRIENDLY COMBINATION: CALCIUM PLUS VITAMIN D

We've known for a long time that taking calcium supplements plus vitamin D can slow bone loss after menopause. Now two important studies—one by French investigators and another by my colleague Bess Dawson-Hughes, M.D., and associates at Tufts—have shown that this combination translates into impressive reductions in hip and other bone fractures. Dr. Dawson-Hughes's investigation followed 389 elderly men and women for three years. About half of the volunteers were given a daily supplement containing 500 milligrams of calcium and 700 international units of vitamin D; the rest received a placebo. During the three years, men and women in the two groups were about equally likely to fall. But only 6 percent of those taking the supplements suffered a fracture, compared with 13 percent of those who were merely getting a placebo. This remarkable benefit is comparable to the effects of hormone replacement therapy and other medications used to treat osteoporosis.

FOLATE

If you've been pregnant any time in the past twenty years, you were probably told to take a vitamin supplement high in folate (also called folic acid), one of the B vitamins. Folate plays a key role in the development of the nervous system; a deficiency during pregnancy increases the risk of nervous system birth defects. More recently we've learned that folate may help prevent heart disease, stroke, and declining mental functioning in the elderly, since it helps control a substance in the blood called homocysteine. (See box.) Also, there's some evidence that low folate intake could be a factor in colon cancer.

It's possible to get adequate folate from the diet, but many women don't consume enough folate-rich foods. Sources include liver, dark green leafy vegetables, broccoli, oranges, beans, and peas. If your diet is low in folate and you decide to take a supplement, 400 micrograms per day is adequate. Select a supplement that also includes 2 milligrams of vitamin B-6 and 2 to 5 micrograms of vitamin B-12, since all three of these nutrients work together.

CORONARY DISEASE: THE HOMOCYSTEINE CONNECTION

When the body processes methionine, an amino acid, one of the byproducts is homocysteine. In order to break it down we need folate, a B vitamin. If we don't get enough, homocysteine may accumulate in the blood. Excessive homocysteine can damage the lining of the arteries, making them more vulnerable to cholesterol deposits.

Attention was drawn to homocysteine more than twenty-five years ago, when a Harvard physician autopsied an 8-year-old boy who had died of a stroke. The child had plaque-choked arteries—and abnormally high homocysteine levels. More recent studies at Tufts by Jacob Selhub, Ph.D., and colleagues found that individuals with elevated amounts of homocysteine in their blood had *triple* the average risk of heart attack. Others have corroborated these findings. Genetic factors appear to affect homocysteine levels. But Dr. Selhub estimates that at least two-thirds of elevated homocysteine can be explained by inadequate intake of folate and of vitamins B-6 and B-12.

VITAMIN C

Vitamin C is a potent antioxidant—indeed, it's sometimes added to food as a preservative—so we've hoped it might act against disease. Dozens of studies have tried to prove that vitamin C can prevent the common cold, but all we know for sure is that it may help shorten the duration and severity of a cold once you've caught it. However, there's persuasive research evidence that vitamin C can help protect against two common causes of vision problems in the elderly: cataracts and macular degeneration. Seven different studies have shown that a daily intake of at least 300 milligrams of vitamin C is associated with a reduction of up to 70 percent in cataracts. It's possible to get 300 milligrams if you eat plenty of fruits and vegetables, which also give you many other nutrients. If you plan to take a vitamin C supplement, I recommend taking between 100 and 200 milligrams per day.

VITAMIN E

This vitamin—found in wheat germ, vegetable oils, and nuts—is another potent antioxidant. Half of Americans don't meet the current RDA for vitamin E, and evidence is accumulating that supplements above the RDA may provide additional health benefits.

My Tufts colleague Simin Meydani, D.V.M., Ph.D., recently published promising findings about vitamin E in the *Journal of the American Medical Association*. She and her associates demonstrated that elderly men and women who took vitamin E supplements for four months showed a 50 percent improvement in several indexes of immune function. Others have found an association between vitamin E supplements and decreased colon cancer, stroke, and Alzheimer's disease. One intriguing English study found that men and women who already suffered from heart disease had 70 percent fewer heart attacks when they took vitamin E. The investigators speculate that oxidized LDLs are the ones most likely to deposit cholesterol in arteries, and that vitamin E prevents them from becoming oxidized. Can vitamin E help younger people too? Possibly, though the benefits seem to be less dramatic. The recommended amount for vitamin E supplementation is 100–200 international units daily.

If you're like most weight-conscious American women, you've probably made many health-promoting changes in your diet already. The food plan in this book will help you make more, not just for the months that you're losing weight but for the rest of your life. Eating well will make you happier, healthier, and more energetic—and you'll look better too.

II

GETTING
STARTED

5

THE SEVEN MENTAL SECRETS OF SUCCESSFUL WEIGHT LOSS

I used to go on a diet every Monday, and also on the first of each month, on January 2 (after our annual New Year's open house), and on the day after my birthday—unless there was cake left over, in which case I'd put it off. There was dieting and there was real life. Until now I had no idea how to make them work together.
       —Alexandra

◆   ◆   ◆

When I was in my twenties I was a competitive marathoner. When I meet a woman who's starting a weight-loss program, I'm struck by how similar her task is to running a marathon. Both require long, hard work despite the fact that the finish line is far away. Success depends on the ability to sustain motivation and focus. That's why weight loss isn't just a matter of diet and exercise. A lot of brainwork is required too.

The mental secrets of successful weight loss aren't really different from the mental secrets of being an athlete, quitting smoking, or taking on any other difficult personal challenge. That's why, when I work with women who want to lose weight, I draw upon seemingly unrelated fields, such as sports psychology and smoking cessation. You probably have most of the necessary mental skills already—if not, you can easily learn them. As you do, you'll find they apply to many areas of your life. When you succeed at losing weight, you will realize that you can succeed at anything.

SECRET #1: BELIEVE THAT YOU CAN DO IT

I'm always concerned when I hear a woman put herself down with statements like these:

> I'm lazy—I'll never be able to exercise.
> I don't have the self-control to follow a food plan.

I believe that we actually listen when we talk to ourselves. Just as we benefit from the supportive words of a loving friend or relative, we need to hear our own encouraging messages. Judith told me:

> I find affirmations very helpful. These are strong, positive statements that I make to myself several times a day. One is: "I am a slender, healthy, energetic, strong, and vibrant woman living my life with grace, ease, and balance." I don't say I wish I could be like this. I say the affirmation as if the changes had already happened.

Believing in yourself really makes a difference. There is dramatic evidence from a 1996 University of Maryland study involving fifty-four women who followed a diet and exercise program for nine months. Before they started, investigators asked them whether they thought they'd lose weight. Twenty-eight of the women were "believers" and twenty-six were "disbelievers." The believers expected to get trim—and they did. At the end of nine months they'd lost 30 percent more weight than those who lacked faith in themselves.

You may feel skeptical. Perhaps you've tried dieting before without results; or you've lost weight only to regain it. Then there's the widely quoted

Becoming a Believer:
The Power of Visualization

These days no serious athlete trains without the help of visualization. You can use the same technique for weight loss. It's easy to learn, simple to do—and remarkably powerful.

Though you can do visualization anywhere, it helps to find a place where you can sit comfortably without being interrupted. Relax, close your eyes, and picture yourself succeeding. Let your mind conjure up as many details as possible. See yourself accomplishing the task step by step.

- **Motivate** yourself by visualizing the changes you're working to achieve.

   I try on my favorite blue suit, which I haven't worn since my pregnancy—and it fits! Wearing the suit, I walk into a meeting at work, aware that I'm standing tall and looking attractive.

- **Prepare** for the day ahead by visualizing what you're going to do.

   I change into walking shoes, and I drink a glass of water. At the park, I move slowly at first, then gradually speed up. I walk briskly along the path, swinging my arms. Afterward, my body feels energized and warm.

- **Troubleshoot** by visualizing yourself managing a difficult situation.

   My sister-in-law serves me a slice of chocolate layer cake. I take one bite, and tell her how delicious it is. Then I put my fork down and talk to my niece. My sister-in-law urges everyone to have seconds. I smile and tell her I'm still enjoying my firsts.

"fact" that more than 90 percent of those who try to take off weight permanently either fail to lose or wind up regaining. It simply isn't true! We now know that this pessimistic prognosis is based mainly on the atypical experience of patients in hospital-based programs. But many people manage to lose weight and keep it off with little or no medical assistance. You probably have lots of friends and relatives who have succeeded. Remember the National Weight Control Registry, which I mentioned in Chapter 2? When scientists from the University of Pittsburgh announced that they wanted to gather information on successful dieters, they had no problem finding hundreds of volunteers.

No matter what happened before, you can lose weight now. Don't be discouraged by earlier efforts. Research on former smokers indicates that it takes four or five tries to finally quit for good. Ninety-one percent of the Weight Control Registry members had tried to lose numerous times before the attempt that finally worked. They eventually succeeded—and you can too.

SECRET #2: TAKE RESPONSIBILITY

I've just urged you to believe that weight loss is possible. Now I want to acknowledge that it definitely is not easy. You may be fighting a sluggish metabolism. You may have a full schedule that leaves no obvious time for exercise. And it's tough to modify lifelong eating habits. Food, unlike smoking, is not something you can just give up. Also, eating isn't merely a biological function; it's part of our social and emotional lives. These are real difficulties, and you deserve lots of credit for resolving to surmount them.

Experts—doctors, nutritionists, trainers, therapists—can offer assistance, as I'll discuss in Chapter 6; friends and family members can provide support. All this is very valuable. But some people look to others for more than just information and encouragement; they're hoping for someone else to *take responsibility*. For instance, a woman may ask her doctor to weigh her every week; or she might tell her husband, "Please stop me if you see me taking seconds." This works for a while—but then her doctor goes on vacation, and she overeats because she doesn't have to worry about her weekly weigh-in. Or she negotiates with her husband for "permission" to take an extra dessert. If she doesn't lose weight, she's not only disappointed for herself, she also feels guilty for letting down the people who are trying to help her—and that's not productive either.

SOMEONE I LOVE NEEDS TO LOSE WEIGHT— WHAT CAN I DO TO HELP?

- ◆ Your husband—whose father died young of heart disease— is overweight and sedentary.

- ◆ Your daughter comes home from junior high in tears because her classmates call her "The Blimp."

- ◆ Your best friend hasn't been able to shake her postpartum depression—and you suspect it's because she's still carrying most of the weight she gained during pregnancy.

It's so hard to see a loved one suffer, and so tempting to try to take charge. Sometimes the other person actually begs you for this kind of assistance. Offer your support—but let them assume responsibility. This expression of confidence is the best way to boost their self-esteem.

- ◆ **Do** help them strategize. **Don't** tell them what to do.

- ◆ **Do** point them to professional help sources if they ask. **Don't** play therapist or nutritionist.

- ◆ **Do** plan nutritious meals; keep wholesome foods on hand for snacks and discard the tempting junk. **Don't** tell them what to eat or what not to eat.

- ◆ **Do** join them for active sports and exercise sessions. **Don't** become a workout cop.

- ◆ **Do** praise their successes. **Don't** criticize them when they slip.

Lean on others at the beginning if you have to, but think of them as the equivalent of training wheels on a bicycle: if you continue to depend on their help, you won't go very far. It's fine to ask a friend to join you for your first few aerobic exercise sessions—but don't skip a workout just because she's not available. The people who succeed at weight loss are the ones who take it upon themselves to change their behavior.

◆ ◆ ◆

My age—44—was sneaking up on me. I felt halfway to 80. I had always been active, but in the last ten years I'd slowed down. I wasn't having fun. Emotionally, I felt I didn't have my life any-more. The only one who could do anything about it was me. I'd been teaching my daughter responsibility. Finally, I told myself to wise up.

—Dianne

◆ ◆ ◆

SECRET #3: SET REALISTIC GOALS

Success provides potent encouragement, even if the achievement is small. So ensure success by setting realistic goals for weight loss.

When I work with a woman who wants to lose weight, one of the first questions I ask her is, "How much do you want to weigh?" It's cause for concern if she gives me a number that's clearly lower than nature intended her to be, a weight that she's never been able to maintain in her entire adult life. When you read Chapter 6, where I discuss weight goals in more detail, you may learn that a healthy weight for you is higher than you thought.

Some people want to drop three dress sizes in eight weeks, or they ex-pect to stick to a very restrictive diet without ever slipping. They may be partly successful, but that's not good enough. So they fail (or think they did), get discouraged, and quit. I recently read a 1997 study from the University of Pennsylvania with a finding that really frustrated me. Investigators recruited sixty significantly overweight women (their average weight was 217 pounds) to participate in a 48-week program. Over the 48 weeks, they lost an average of 35 pounds, nearly a pound a week. That's a terrific accomplishment! These women should have been thrilled—but many were disappointed because they'd hoped to lose a lot more.

By coincidence, on the same day I saw that report, I read a delightful message from Nancy, a member of the group that tested the program in this book. Like the women in the University of Pennsylvania study, Nancy has lost slightly under a pound a week. But what a difference in her attitude:

> *Good news: I have lost another three pounds to make a total of nineteen pounds in the past six months. I've also been running/walking two miles almost every day. At first I could only run about a third of the distance, and walked the rest. Now I can run for about three-quarters of it. And yesterday, though I really didn't have the time, I jumped into the swimming pool afterward and swam three laps. I feel wonderful and full of energy!*

I find that the women most likely to succeed in losing weight are the ones whose chief motivation is to become healthier. They measure their progress not only at the scale but also against fitness goals. Of course, they're pleased to look better; however, they consider this a happy extra. Women whose aim is to fit into a bikini often wind up frustrated by slow weight loss, because they feel they've achieved nothing until they reach their goal. There's a risk they'll push themselves too hard—exercise excessively, restrict their eating too much—and burn out.

I've been discussing your long-term aims, but intermediate goals are important too. It can be overwhelming to look ahead to everything you want to accomplish. If you focus instead on smaller weekly aims, they seem doable. Achieving these goals is very reinforcing, and makes the next week much easier. Nancy told me:

> *I play games with myself. It's a challenge to see how far I can run. I used to have to stop twice between my house and a particular road. Now I can run all the way, and that makes me feel good.*

Weight loss should be a very positive experience. You're doing something important for yourself—not only becoming slimmer, but also gaining all the benefits of exercise and good nutrition. These improvements happen quickly, even with slow, sensible weight loss. If you enjoy them, you'll reap the rewards of this program much sooner, and your enthusiasm will remain high.

♦ ♦ ♦

I've lost forty-six pounds over a twelve-month period, and still have a long way to go. But this is not like waiting for a package to be delivered, where you have nothing until it finally arrives. Yes, I'm still overweight—but I'm already stronger, and I have much more stamina and flexibility. No, I'm not slender. But I look better, and I fit into clothes I haven't been able to wear for years.
    —Alexandra

♦ ♦ ♦

SECRET #4: MAKE A FIRM COMMITMENT NOW

Think how you make a vacation happen. You don't wait for a time when your schedule is completely empty for two weeks. If you did that, you'd never get a vacation. Instead you pick the dates and make reservations. Suddenly the trip fits into your life—because you make it fit. You switch appointments to clear your calendar; you let friends and colleagues know that you'll be out of town; you arrange for a neighbor to feed the cats and pick up the mail. Pretty soon you're on your way.

You've already taken an important first step toward losing weight: you're reading this book. The second step is to make the decision to follow the program. Some people get stuck at this point:

I definitely want to try it.
Maybe I'll begin after the holidays.
I'll ask my sister if she wants to do it with me.
One of these days I'll be ready.

Procrastination has insidious effects. Your enthusiasm cools off; your motivation dissolves. You begin to feel guilty about the delay, so you avoid thinking about plans. It becomes increasingly difficult to overcome the inertia.

I urge you to take advantage of your current interest. Assume that you *will* begin strength training and aerobic exercise, that you *will* follow the food plan. Then begin to act on that assumption. Follow the step-by-step instructions in Chapter 10. Buy the weights, select an aerobic activity, plan menus, and stock up on wholesome foods. Then your healthy new lifestyle will begin.

SECRET #5: PLAN FOR SUCCESS

My schedule is normally very hectic. In addition to a demanding job, I have a husband and three young children. Usually I find the pressure stimulating. But a couple of months ago I took on a few new obligations, then found myself getting frazzled. My tension level increased and my productivity sank.

When I realized what was happening, I made time to sit down and get organized. This made all the difference. As soon as I wrote down my obligations, they stopped crashing around in my head causing friction. I divided big jobs into small, doable pieces. Tasks that had seemed enormous suddenly shrank. I went through my calendar and figured out when everything would get done. This planning session took about fifteen minutes, but my increased efficiency gave me many hours—and dramatically reduced my stress.

You're about to create significant changes in your life. You'll make decisions about food and exercise; you'll buy equipment and supplies. There will be new skills to learn and new activities to fit into your schedule. That's a lot to tackle at once, even with help from this book. Planning will help you sort everything out so the pieces fall into place. Once you get going, planning will help you continue.

Barbara, a working mother with five children, describes how she set up a weekly routine for exercise:

> *The best time for me to swim is late afternoon, before dinner, when I'm sluggish. I swim on Sundays, Mondays, and Thursdays between four and six o'clock. I try to avoid scheduling appointments at those times, but if it can't be helped, I substitute a Tuesday swim. This way, I'm never afraid of finding out on Saturday that a week has gone by and I haven't exercised.*

Built-in flexibility is an important part of Barbara's plan. It wouldn't work if she couldn't adapt to unexpected demands on her time.

Planning is more than a management strategy; it's a way of nurturing yourself, as Sarah points out:

> *This may sound trivial, but one of the nicest things I do for myself is to prepare fruit. I cut up a melon after a meal, when I'm not hungry—and later, when I need an instant snack, there it is. I peel and section an orange in the evening—and as if by magic, a ready-to-eat orange is waiting for me in the morning, when I'm still half asleep.*

SECRET #6: KEEP RECORDS

Kaiser Permanente, one of the country's largest HMOs, was running a weight-loss program with more than 2,000 participants, and the program leaders wanted to learn what factors were associated with success. They looked at age, activity level, starting weight, and many other variables. What was the best predictor? The answer may surprise you: keeping food records. Other studies have corroborated this finding. Indeed, research has shown that people who simply keep food records lose weight, even when they don't consciously eat less. Similar research has found the same for exercise: people who keep logs stick with their exercise programs.

What makes records so effective? We don't know for sure, but here are some possibilities:

♦ Record-keeping reflects characteristics that make for success: strong motivation; attention to program requirements.

♦ Records help you follow a food or exercise plan, because they keep track of details. For instance, if you tally the day's food allotment, you'll know if you're eating enough fruit, or if you can take an extra snack without going over.

When you write down the dumbbells you lift for each exercise, you know which ones to use the next time. This makes your workouts more efficient.

◆ Records are a constant reminder of your commitment. I often hear comments like this: *I was tempted to take seconds, but I resisted because I didn't want to write it down.*

◆ Over time, records help you see how far you've come. That's very motivating. If you've been sedentary, you may struggle during your first ten-minute aerobics session. Write that down—and read it in a month or two, when you're able to sustain twenty or thirty minutes.

You might think that it takes complicated records to be effective. Not so. Simply checking off boxes on a form—such as those in Chapter 10—makes a big difference. Some people actually like to keep detailed food or exercise logs. They write down exactly what they eat at every meal or snack, and they have similar descriptions of their workouts. That's fine, but most women prefer minimal record-keeping.

Members of the group that tested the program in this book recognized the benefit of recording their workouts. They soon discovered that if they didn't write down the weights they lifted for the arm exercises, they'd forget at least one of them by the next session. Some also took to food logs; but others were considerably less enthusiastic, even though I pointed out that the forms required less than two minutes a day.

I told them: "Some people can stay on track without food records, and it's fine for them to skip this step. However, if you find that you're not doing as well with the food plan as you'd hoped, I urge you to give record-keeping a try—you'll be amazed at how potent it is."

SECRET #7: REBOUND—
AND LEARN—FROM MISTAKES

If you watch the Olympics, you've seen dramas like this: a figure skater is per-forming a complex program, the culmination of years of training. She stum-bles badly in her first jump, losing points. But despite this confidence-shaking disappointment, she completes the rest of her routine flawlessly and wins.

Learning how to bounce back and persevere is one of the most helpful lessons I've learned from sports psychology, and it's invaluable for many as-pects of life, including weight loss. Setbacks are inevitable in any long-term effort. Yet some people become so distracted and demoralized by small fail-ures that they forget their larger successes and go off track. As a result, a prob-lem that should have been small and temporary becomes large and persistent. Remember the University of Maryland study I mentioned earlier, the one that found people who believed in themselves were more successful at weight loss? I think it's significant that the believers were not only more self-confident, they were also less likely than the disbelievers to berate themselves for mis-takes—showing the power of the language you use with yourself.

If you overeat on Thanksgiving, you might gain a pound or two. That's of little long-term consequence, provided you return to your food plan right away. Here's what sports psychologists tell athletes—I think it's great advice for everyone:

- Don't be self-critical just because you've made an error. Mistakes are unfortunate, but they're a normal part of life. That's why almost all pencils come with built-in erasers.

- Look back only to learn from what happened, not to criti-cize yourself. After you've extracted the lessons, move on.

- Concentrate on the task ahead.

- Remind yourself how far you've come toward your long-term goals. You've got a lot to be proud of!

WHAT HAVE YOU GOT
TO LOSE?

When you're a teenager, you learn all these rules from your girl-friends: if you stand with your knees touching, there should be a space between your thighs. Your waist should be ten inches smaller than your hips and chest. You should weigh 100 pounds plus five pounds for each inch over five feet. Even though you grow up and realize how dumb these rules are, they remain stuck somewhere in your brain.

—Alexandra

◆   ◆   ◆

As you begin this program and set goals for yourself, you're probably wondering how much you should weigh. That's a very good question, but I can't provide a simple answer. I'll start by giving you the same suggestion I give to the women I work with: if you have a particular weight in mind, set it aside for a moment so you can take a fresh look. What's important really isn't a specific number on a scale, but looking good, being healthy, and feeling vibrant and fit. Moreover, your aims need to be tempered with realism. If you try to become thinner than you've ever been in your adult life, you'll have to struggle to achieve and maintain the lower weight.

In addition to thinking about your goals, you'll need to decide if you should see a doctor or arrange for other assistance before you begin. This chapter will help you through these preliminaries—and then you'll be ready to start.

◆ ◆ ◆

I have an 11-year-old daughter. I want her to be strong, to exercise, and to eat well, so she'll be confident and feel really good about herself. And I want her to do all these things for healthy reasons, without worrying about what she looks like. So I'm trying to be a good role model for her.
    —Therese

◆ ◆ ◆

THAT MAGIC NUMBER

When I talk to women about their weight goals, many of them admit that they're still fixed on a number—a weight or a dress size—left over from their teenage years. Because that magic number represents being attractive and slender, it carries a lot of emotional baggage. Jill told me:

I wanted to be like Margot Fonteyn: 5 feet 4 inches, 114 pounds. Today, that would be heavy for a ballet dancer. The trouble was, I reached 5 feet 4 inches at age 13 and kept going. But I still remember 114 pounds.

Jill agreed to set aside this number and rethink her goals. I asked about her weight history. She's 5 feet 6 inches tall and—except for a period of depression which she gained 20 pounds—she's weighed between 135 and 140. Recently the scale has crept into the 140 to 145 pound range, which concerns her. Despite the fact that she eats well and does aerobic exercise, her clothes are getting snug.

Many women don't set weight goals when they start this program. They simply want to get healthier and fitter—and that's absolutely fine. But others, like Jill, want a specific objective. If that's your preference, I believe that three factors are important in coming up with your goal:

- **What's healthy** should be your primary concern—feeling good, physically and emotionally. Later in this chapter I'll explain how to determine a healthy weight range for your height. Jill was surprised to learn how wide this range is—in her case, 118 to 155 pounds. She'd felt sluggish, bloated, and unattractive during the brief period that she weighed 155, so that was not a good weight for her.

- **What's realistic** must be carefully considered too. The best indicator is your own history. True, 118 or even 114 pounds wouldn't be an unhealthy weight for Jill, but is it realistic? Her normal eating and exercise habits—which had kept her at 135 to 140 pounds for years—would need to be changed significantly. A woman whose weight or sedentary lifestyle put her at risk for serious health problems has compelling reasons to make major changes. But that wasn't true for Jill.

- **What it takes to look your best** is important—but this is not simply a matter of what you weigh. When you eat well and become fit, you naturally look better. Strength training trims and tightens, so you're slimmer even if you don't shed a pound. After a few weeks of nutritious eating and good hydration, women whose diet had been haphazard often notice improvements in their appearance: their skin is no longer dry; their hair becomes glossy. Increased self-confidence and energy also do wonders for a person's looks.

A woman who's overweight and unhappy about her appearance sometimes feels that losing weight is the only answer. But there's so much more she can do to look better. I'm sure you've seen makeovers in magazines and on TV, with startlingly different "before" and "after" pictures. The woman is transformed not because she's lost weight, but because she has a new haircut, touches of makeup, new glasses, and well-chosen clothes—and it doesn't hurt that she's smiling happily and standing tall.

Jill realized that her previously normal weight range, 135 to 140 pounds, was probably best for her. By slightly increasing her aerobic activity and cutting back a little on snacks, she should be able to get there in about ten weeks. Because she's started strength training, I won't be surprised if she's a size smaller this time than she previously was at that weight. As you read through this chapter, I hope you'll rethink your goals. Most women tell me they feel liberated and unencumbered when they're finally able to unload the unrealistic and burdensome numbers they've carried for years.

◆ ◆ ◆

A woman in my weight-loss class said that her ideal weight was based on a Barbie doll she had when she was a girl. It came with a scale. Barbie was supposed to be 5 foot 9 and the number painted on the scale was 110 pounds. That brought home to me the unrealistic goals that people set for themselves.
—Isabel

◆ ◆ ◆

WHAT'S THE BEST WEIGHT FOR YOUR HEALTH?

Remember those old scales where you put in a penny and got your weight and fortune? Printed on top was the Metropolitan Life Insurance Company's table of ideal body weights for men and women, by height. Metropolitan Life had gathered data about their customers for decades, and the tables represented what they'd learned about the optimal weights for longevity and health. Their height-weight tables were widely used—you may have seen them in books and magazines or at your doctor's office—but they simply created two categories: ideal and everything else. Obviously, the degree of overweight matters too. So these days, experts use the Body Mass Index (BMI) instead of the Metropolitan Life tables. The underlying information, which comes from insurance company statistics and large-scale health studies, is really the same. However, the BMI combines height and weight into a single number—the higher above normal it is, the greater the health risks.

Body Mass Index (For Women and Men)

1. Read down the first column to locate your height.
2. Read across that row and locate your weight.
3. Read the heading on top of the column—that's your BMI.

Height (inches)	18	19	20	21	22	23	24	25	26	27	28	29	30	31	32	33	34	35	36	37	38	39	40 or more
58	86	91	96	100	105	110	115	119	124	129	134	138	143	148	153	158	162	167	172	177	181	186	191+
59	89	94	99	104	109	114	119	124	128	133	138	143	148	153	158	163	168	173	178	183	188	193	198+
60	92	97	102	107	112	118	123	128	133	138	143	148	153	158	163	168	174	179	184	189	194	199	204+
61	95	100	106	111	116	122	127	132	137	143	148	153	158	164	169	174	180	185	190	195	201	206	211+
62	98	104	109	115	120	126	131	136	142	147	153	158	164	169	175	180	186	191	196	202	207	213	218+
63	101	107	113	118	124	130	135	141	146	152	158	163	169	175	180	186	191	197	203	208	214	220	225+
64	105	110	116	122	128	134	140	145	151	157	163	169	174	180	186	192	197	204	209	215	221	227	232+
65	108	114	120	126	132	138	144	150	156	162	168	174	180	186	192	198	204	210	216	222	228	234	240+
66	111	118	124	130	136	142	148	155	161	167	173	179	186	192	198	204	210	216	223	229	235	241	247+
67	115	121	127	134	140	146	153	159	166	172	178	185	191	198	204	211	217	223	230	236	242	249	255+
68	118	125	131	138	144	151	158	164	171	177	184	190	197	203	210	216	223	230	236	243	249	256	262+
69	122	128	135	142	149	155	162	169	176	182	189	196	203	209	216	223	230	236	243	250	257	263	270+
70	125	132	139	146	153	160	167	174	181	188	195	202	209	216	223	229	236	243	250	257	264	271	278+
71	129	136	143	150	157	165	172	179	186	193	200	208	215	222	229	236	243	250	257	265	272	279	286+
72	132	140	147	154	162	169	177	184	191	199	206	213	221	228	235	242	250	258	265	272	279	287	294+

BMI under 19: Underweight
BMI 19 to 25: Healthy weight
BMI 26 to 30: Overweight

BMI 31 to 39: Very overweight
BMI 40 and above: Extremely overweight

How to Calculate Your BMI

(Or Where to Go on the Internet to Have the Calculation Done for You)

Here's a three-step method for computing your BMI if you know your weight and height. A calculator will help.

Step 1: Multiply your weight in pounds by 703.

Step 2: Multiply your height in inches by itself.

Step 3: Divide the first number by the second.

Round to the nearest whole number—that's your BMI.

Example: Gretchen weighs 180 pounds; she's 5 feet, 5 inches (65 inches) tall.

Step 1: $180 \times 703 = 126{,}540$

Step 2: $65 \times 65 = 4{,}225$

Step 3: $126{,}540 \div 4{,}225 = 29.95$

Gretchen's BMI is 30.

The Web site of *Shape Up America!*—a superb fitness and nutrition education program initiated by former U.S. Surgeon General Dr. C. Everett Koop—has BMI tables and information. If you provide your height and weight, you can learn your BMI instantly. The URL is: http://www.shapeup.org.

THE BODY MASS INDEX

Your BMI is your weight in kilograms divided by the square of your height, in meters—but don't sharpen your pencil yet! The simplest way to determine your BMI is to look it up on a chart (see page 91). Another way is to use the instructions on this page to do the calculation in pounds and inches.

WHAT'S YOUR BMI?

If you've recently had your weight and height measured on a medical visit, use those numbers. Otherwise start by weighing yourself in the morning, before you eat breakfast. Since the charts are based on weights without clothing, wear as little as possible.

Next, measure your height. You can do this yourself, but it's easier if someone helps you. Stand in bare feet with your back to a wall. Your heels should be against the wall; your head should be held high but not tilted back. Rest a ruler flat on top of your head, keeping it parallel to the floor. Mark the spot where the ruler touches the wall. Then measure the wall from floor to mark to determine your height.

If you're over age 40, it's a good idea to measure your height at least once a year. Getting shorter could be a sign of osteoporosis. If you discover that you've shrunk more than an inch (anything less could simply reflect a measurement error), tell your doctor.

Now, find your BMI on the chart on page 91.

HOW TO INTERPRET YOUR BMI

Your BMI tells you whether your weight falls into a range that's optimal for longevity and good health. However, I want to emphasize that you're an individual, not a statistic. Weight, though important, is just one factor in determining your risk of disease—lifestyle, family history, and current health also matter. For instance, if you're overweight but fit and healthy, you're at much lower risk for heart disease than someone who has the same BMI or even lower but who's sedentary and suffering from diabetes.

BMI Under 19: Underweight

Because overweight is such a prevalent problem, we sometimes forget that it's not healthy to be underweight either. A BMI under 19 is associated with elevated risk for cancer, osteoporosis, and infertility. It can also be a sign of emotional problems, including anxiety, depression, suicidal tendencies, and sleep difficulties. Since emotional problems may be tied to eating disorders, which can be life-threatening, it's very important to seek diagnosis and appropriate treatment. (See box on eating disorders on page 94.)

If your BMI is below 19, you should not attempt to lose weight. However, you can use the *Strong Women Stay Slim* program to become fitter and to develop healthier eating patterns. I often see women who are underweight but over-fat—they're thin but not toned. If your body is like that, you cer-

MIGHT YOU HAVE AN EATING DISORDER?

Women with eating disorders come in all different sizes, from thin to heavy. The following statements are adapted from material developed by Anorexia Nervosa and Related Eating Disorders, Inc. The more items that apply to you, the more serious your problem may be—and the more important it is for you to seek help.

- Even though my doctor and my friends tell me I'm thin, I feel fat.

- Other people worry about the way I eat; I lie about my eating.

- When I eat, I'm afraid I won't be able to stop.

- I feel guilty when I eat.

- I have missed work or school because of my weight or eating habits.

- When I eat, I feel bloated and fat.

- I do strange things with my food—for example, cut it into tiny pieces, eat it on special dishes with special utensils, make patterns on my plate with it, secretly spit it out.

- To control my weight, I vomit, take laxatives or diuretics, or fast.

- I get anxious if I can't exercise.

- I have said or thought, "I would rather die than be fat."

- I have noticed one or more of the following: irregular or absent menstrual periods (even though I'm premenopausal), cold hands and feet, dry skin, thinning hair, fragile nails, swollen glands in my neck, dental cavities, dizziness, weakness, fainting, rapid or irregular heartbeat.

For referrals and further information about eating disorders:

ANOREXIA NERVOSA AND RELATED EATING DISORDERS, INC.
P.O. Box 5102
Eugene, OR 97405
Tel: 541-344-1144
http://www.ANRED.com

NATIONAL EATING DISORDERS ORGANIZATION
6655 South Yale Avenue
Tulsa, OK 74136
Tel: 918-481-4044

NATIONAL ASSOCIATION OF ANOREXIA NERVOSA
AND ASSOCIATED DISORDERS
P.O. Box 7
Highland Park, IL 60035
Tel: 847-831-3438

EATING DISORDER AWARENESS AND PREVENTION, INC.
603 Stewart Street, Suite 803
Seattle, WA 98101
Tel: 206-382-3587
http://members.aol.com/edapinc

tainly don't need to lose weight, but you could benefit by trading some of your fat for muscle. Strengthening exercise and aerobics will make you stronger, firmer, and shapelier. You might also consider trying to slowly gain a few pounds so that your weight falls into the "healthy" BMI category.

BMI Between 19 and 25: Healthy Weight

This BMI range is associated with the longest life and lowest risk for disease. The range is wider than you might expect, because it covers men as well as women, and people of all ages and different builds. I realize that some women in this category are not happy with their weight while others are perfectly content.

WHAT'S YOUR WAIST-TO-HIP RATIO?

Excess fat around the abdomen—a high waist-to-hip ratio—is strongly associated with **Syndrome X,** a cluster of symptoms that signal elevated risk for both heart disease and diabetes: high blood pressure, resistance to insulin, and high levels of cholesterol and other fat in the blood. This is why doctors are more concerned when an overweight person has a large belly rather than big hips and thighs.

Are you at risk for Syndrome X? To find out, first measure your waist. Some people have an obvious waistline. If yours isn't clear, find the smallest circumference between the upper part of your hipbone and the lowest part of your rib cage on your side, and measure that. The tape should be neither tight nor loose. Women are at elevated risk if their waist is 35 inches or larger.

If your waist is less than 35 inches, you'll need to calculate your waist-to-hip ratio to assess your risk. Measure the widest point on your hips. Then divide your waist measurement by your hip measurement.

- ♦ **Favorable**: Waist-to-hip ratio less than .80

- ♦ **Borderline**: Waist-to-hip ratio between .80 and .85

- ♦ **Unfavorable**: Waist-to-hip ratio above .85, or waist 35 inches or larger

Though there's a strong genetic component to body shape, aerobic exercise and weight loss can decrease waist size and the waist-to-hip ratio.

What's a reasonable goal for you? Ask yourself these questions:

- ♦ **Are you at above-average risk for heart disease or diabetes?** If so, I'd suggest you aim for a BMI at the mid to low end of the healthy range.

◆ **What's your weight history?** If you know you feel and look better at the mid to low end of the healthy range, that's a good goal. However, I don't recommend you aim for a weight you've never been able to sustain. Instead, concentrate on going down one or two BMI points, while eating well and becoming fit. At that point, if you're still not satisfied, you can always lose some more.

◆ **Are you unhappy about your appearance?** As you start to eat better and exercise more, you will undoubtedly see improvements—and possibly a difference on the scale as well. Most women who follow this program find that they're satisfied with themselves at a heavier weight than they would have expected.

BMI Between 26 and 30: Moderately Overweight
BMI Between 31 and 39: Very Overweight
BMI 40 and up: Extremely Overweight

The higher your BMI, the greater the risk that you'll suffer from weight-related disability or disease. Individuals with a BMI of 40 and over are at substantial risk. The danger is further increased if you have a high waist-to-hip ratio (see box on page 96) and additional risk factors, such as high blood pressure or elevated blood cholesterol or blood sugar.

If you are in any of these three BMI categories, I suggest that you set as an initial goal losing enough weight to move down two BMI numbers. This change has been shown to improve health, especially if accomplished with increased physical activity and improved nutrition. If you have any of the additional risk factors mentioned above, you should see an effect on them too. As a longer-term goal, try to bring yourself down to the next lower BMI category. If you're already suffering from weight-related illness or disability, the change probably will make a big difference in your symptoms.

Don't be discouraged if you have a long way to go. You'll see significant improvements very quickly, even if you're still overweight. As you progress, you'll feel and look better. And with each lower BMI number, your health risks are reduced. Think of two BMI numbers as a stepping-stone, and focus on moving down just one step at a time.

Physical Activity Readiness
Questionnaire—PAR-Q
(revised 1994)

PAR-Q & YOU
(A Questionnaire for People Aged 15 to 69)

Regular physical activity is fun and healthy, and increasingly more people are starting to become more active every day. Being more active is very safe for most people. However, some people should check with their doctor before they start becoming much more physically active.

If you are planning to become much more physically active than you are now, start by answering the seven questions in the box below. If you are between the ages of 15 and 69, the PAR-Q will tell you if you should check with your doctor before you start. If you are over 69 years of age, and you are not used to being very active, check with your doctor.

Common sense is your best guide when you answer these questions. Please read the questions carefully and answer each one honestly: check YES or NO.

YES NO

☐ ☐ 1. Has your doctor ever said that you have a heart condition <u>and</u> that you should only do physical activity recommended by a doctor?

☐ ☐ 2. Do you feel pain in your chest when you do physical activity?

☐ ☐ 3. In the past month, have you had chest pain when you were not doing physical activity?

☐ ☐ 4. Do you lose your balance because of dizziness or do you ever lose consciousness?

☐ ☐ 5. Do you have a bone or joint problem that could be made worse by a change in your physical activity?

☐ ☐ 6. Is your doctor currently prescribing drugs (for example, water pills) for your blood pressure or heart condition?

☐ ☐ 7. Do you know of <u>any other reason</u> why you should not do physical activity?

IF YOU ANSWERED

YES to one or more questions

Talk with your doctor by phone or in person BEFORE you start becoming much more physically active or BEFORE you have a fitness appraisal. Tell your doctor about the PAR-Q and which questions you answered YES.

- ♦ You may be able to do any activity you want—as long as you start slowly and build up gradually. Or, you may need to restrict your activities to those which are safe for you. Talk with your doctor about the kinds of physical activities you wish to participate in and follow his/her advice.
- ♦ Find out which community programs are safe and helpful for you.

NO to all questions

If you answered NO honestly to *all* PAR-Q questions, you can be reasonably sure that you can:

- ♦ start becoming much more physically active—begin slowly and build up gradually. This is the safest and easiest way to go.
- ♦ take part in a fitness appraisal—this is an excellent way to determine your basic fitness so that you can plan the best way for you to live actively.

DELAY BECOMING MUCH MORE ACTIVE:

- ♦ if you are not feeling well because of a temporary illness such as a cold or fever—wait until you feel better; or
- ♦ if you are or may be pregnant—talk to your doctor before you start becoming more active.

Please note: If your health changes so that you then answer YES to any of the above questions, tell your fitness or health professional. Ask whether you should change your physical activity plan.

Informed Use of the PAR-Q: The Canadian Society for Exercise Physiology, Health Canada, and their agents assume no liability for persons who undertake physical activity, and if in doubt after completing this questionnaire, consult your doctor prior to physical activity.

Reprinted by special permission from the Canadian Society for Exercise Physiology, Inc., copyright © 1994, SCEP.

DO YOU NEED TO SEE YOUR DOCTOR?

Many women skip medical checkups. They're busy; they're feeling fine and don't see the need; they worry about the expense or fear bad news. If you haven't had a checkup for a year or more, please make an appointment. Routine physical examinations can detect cancer and other serious medical problems long before symptoms appear, when treatment is most effective.

Overweight women may avoid the doctor out of embarrassment, or because they expect criticism. If such concerns have held you back in the past, I hope you feel more confident now that you're starting this program. A supportive doctor will discuss diet and exercise strategies, and take baseline measurements—such as weight, blood pressure, blood cholesterol, and blood sugar—that will help you track your progress. If your doctor isn't helpful, don't be shy about expressing your concern and asking for what you need. If you aren't satisfied with the response, consider seeking another physician.

BEFORE YOU TRY TO LOSE WEIGHT

Your doctor may have already told you that losing weight is not only safe but also highly desirable. However, some women have physical conditions that make weight loss inappropriate, even if they're currently overweight. For example, losing weight is not advised during pregnancy. If you have any chronic medical condition—including Parkinson's disease, multiple sclerosis, or rheumatoid arthritis—discuss your weight goals with your doctor before starting this program.

BEFORE YOU CHANGE YOUR DIET

The food plan in this program follows well-established nutrition guidelines for healthy Americans. However, some individuals will need to modify it. Discuss the diet with your doctor if you're pregnant or breastfeeding, or if you follow a therapeutic diet for a medical condition, such as diabetes or kidney disease.

BEFORE YOU BEGIN EXERCISING

The exercise programs in this book are safe for nearly everyone. However, some women should talk to a doctor before increasing their physical activity. Take the PAR-Q—Physical Activity Readiness Questionnaire—to see if this caution applies to you. Remember, if you're in doubt, err on the side of safety and check with your doctor.

COULD YOU USE SOME EXTRA HELP?

I've tried to make this book as comprehensive as possible, but you may know from past experience that you'll need extra support. Working one-on-one with a professional can make a big difference—and it may not be as costly as you'd expect. Many medical insurance plans and HMOs cover classes and individual consultations for people trying to lose weight; some offer discounted rates at local fitness centers. More and more employers provide this kind of help as well. It's really not surprising: exercise and weight loss are so beneficial to health that insurers and employers actually save money in the long run by paying for such support. Even if you have to bear the cost of professional assistance and are limited in what you can afford, a few sessions could be very valuable, especially when you're getting started or if you run into problems later on.

Useful help sources include:

NUTRITIONISTS

My family won't eat "diet food" and I don't have time to cook separate meals.
Menu planning is a problem for me.
When I go on a diet, I'm hungry all the time.

The food plan in this book is a healthy way of eating that will benefit every member of your family. But they may take a little convincing. A nutritionist could help you devise menus that match your family's preferences (and yours).

The initials R.D., which stand for Registered Dietitian, mean that a nutritionist has met the stringent requirements of the American Dietetic Association. To find an R.D. in your area, ask your health-care provider or contact the American Dietetic Association at 800-366-1655 or at http://www.eatright.org.

EXERCISE TRAINERS

I find it hard to follow instructions from a book.
I've got a bad elbow, so I worry about doing some of the exercises.
I'd like some moves to address my "love handles."

Although most people won't need a trainer to learn the exercises in this book, others do better with extra assistance. A trainer can help you learn the moves and proper form for strength-training exercises and aerobic workouts. As you progress, the trainer can recheck your form, answer questions, and offer encouragement. When you're ready to make changes—such as expanding your strength-training program or beginning a new kind of aerobic exercise—the trainer can advise you.

Many exercise class instructors see clients privately. Get a referral from a local health club (even if you're not a member), or call an adult education program. Make sure the trainer has experience working with people like you, especially if you have special concerns or unusual needs. The trainer should have certification from at least one of the following organizations: the American College of Sports Medicine; the National Strength and Conditioning Association; the National Academy of Sports Medicine; the American Council on Exercise; Aerobics and Fitness Association of America; IDEA—the International Association of Fitness Professionals; or the Cooper Institute for Aerobics Research.

◆　◆　◆

When I began strength training I worked with a trainer because I have a tendency to get hurt. I have chronic back pain from a tennis injury I got more than twenty years ago. The trainer taught me strengthening exercises for my upper and lower body, and also suggested limbering exercises. She told me to stop doing an exercise I was using for back pain—and my back got better. When I had a flare-up, she helped me modify my workouts.
　　—Judith

◆　◆　◆

PSYCHOTHERAPISTS

My eating is so out of control that it scares me sometimes.
When I lose weight and begin to look different, I become anxious
and depressed and I start overeating again.
Other people undermine my efforts if I try to lose weight: my hus-
band complains about the time I spend exercising; my mother says
I'm too thin; my best friend says I'm no fun anymore. I don't know
how to cope with this.

Sometimes women gain weight because they're going through a trou-
bled period; for other women, eating and weight become so entangled with
emotion that change is difficult. Once they get help, it's easier to follow a program of sensible eating and exercise—and often many other aspects of their
lives improve as well.

Consider seeking psychological assistance when you suspect that
deeper emotional issues are getting in your way. Try to find a therapist who
specializes in weight-related problems. This is especially important if you suspect that you might have an eating disorder. Good referral sources are your
doctor, or the psychology, psychiatry, or clinical nutrition department at a local teaching hospital; the organizations listed in the box about eating disorders (page 95) also provide referrals.

SUPPORT GROUPS

I need lots of encouragement, but my family and friends get tired
of hearing about my diet.
It really inspires me to see "Before" and "After" pictures of people
who've lost weight.
For me, the best advice comes from other women who are doing
the same thing.

Weight-loss support groups provide companionship and inspiration,
plus a ready source of helpful tips. As you get slimmer and fitter, you'll have
the satisfaction of serving as a model for others.

Your health-care provider probably can refer you to a group; commercial and self-help weight-control organizations are listed in the telephone Yellow Pages under "Reducing" or "Weight Reduction." Groups vary, even within
the same organization, so check out others if you don't care for the first one

you try. Another option is an online support group. If you subscribe to AOL, begin with Keyword DIET; on CompuServe, use Go GOODDIET; on the Internet, visit http://www.diettalk.com.

◆ ◆ ◆

I'm good at networking. I get a lot of support by talking to people and sharing ideas. A core group of people in my diet group showed up every week. What we liked most was talking about strategies—practical, usable stuff: How do you deal with eating at a restaurant? What are your techniques for not eating when something is seducing you? How do you manage at parties?
—Therese

◆ ◆ ◆

If you need more than one kind of help, call your HMO or a local teaching hospital. Many have excellent weight-reduction programs that offer multiple resources, including doctors, nutritionists, exercise physiologists, psychologists, and support groups.

III

THE STRONG WOMEN STAY SLIM PROGRAM

▼   ▼   ▼   ▼

7

SIX EXERCISES THAT WILL MAKE YOU STRONG

I can run upstairs without my knees killing me for the first time in many years. I'm a professional violinist, and I'm finding that my increased upper body strength has been a real boost to my endurance during long performances—an unexpected bonus! And all of this after only a few weeks of strength training.
        —Sue

◆   ◆   ◆

Strength training is the foundation of the *Strong Women Stay Slim* weight-loss program. The exercise plan outlined in this chapter requires just three twenty-minute sessions per week, but it produces extraordinary effects. The major muscle groups in your body—your arms, shoulders, back, abdomen, buttocks, and legs—will become significantly stronger. Strength training is exciting because you notice improvements in a few weeks. That's around the time you begin aerobic activity. And behind the scenes, these exercises build muscle and bone tissue, so your body gets leaner and healthier as you lose weight.

The key to success with strength training is to start at an easy level and work up slowly but steadily. I'll explain exactly how to customize the program to give you the right challenge. This chapter also includes two extra strengthening exercises that you can incorporate after a month or two, when you're ready for more.

GEAR

To strengthen your muscles, you have to work them harder than usual. Four of the exercises use dumbbells. The others use your own body weight: by changing position, you can increase or decrease the load on your muscles. You don't have to join a gym, buy costly weight machines, or purchase ankle cuffs. All you need are dumbbells and a container or rack to hold them, plus a few simple items you probably have around the house.

DUMBBELLS

During the first week, most women do the exercises with 1-pound weights. But you'll move up very quickly, and eventually go past 10 pounds for most of the arm exercises.

Dumbbells can be purchased in 1-pound increments. While a complete set is really best, it's expensive and takes up a lot of space. So here's my suggestion for a workable compromise between convenience and cost:

◆ Instead of starting with 1-pound dumbbells—which you'll probably use only the first week—do the exercises holding a 1-pound can in each hand. Select tall, narrow cans rather than short, wide ones, so you can hold them securely. Note: I do not recommend using larger cans when you graduate to heavier weights, because they're too big to grip safely.

◆ Buy pairs of dumbbells in 3-, 5-, 6-, 8- and 10-pound weights. A suggestion for economizing: check out the sets of dumbbells sold by many sporting goods stores; buying a set and filling in the missing weights may save you money.

◆ To keep initial costs down, don't buy heavier weights immediately. Wait until you've progressed to 10-pound weights on some of the exercises. At that point, women typically need 12- and 15-pound dumbbells to get the most out of the program.

You can also save money by sharing weights with friends, or buying used dumbbells. For safety's sake, I don't recommend improvising equipment from water jugs or buckets; they're not designed for strength training and could be unsafe. The small investment required for good equipment makes sense—after all, you're spending your valuable time on these workouts.

Dumbbells up to 10 pounds are sold in discount and department stores, as well as in shops that sell sporting equipment. However, for heavier dumbbells, you'll probably need a specialty store. Check the Yellow Pages under "Sporting Goods" to find shops near you, and call to make sure they have what you require.

Some women prefer to mail-order their weights, not only for shopping convenience but to avoid transporting them home. (Note: shipping costs make this option much more expensive.) Here are some sources:

FITNESS DISTRIBUTORS
25 Washington Street
Natick, MA 01760
Tel: 800-244-1882 or 508-653-1882
Fax: 508-650-0448

MC SPORTS
3070 Shaffer Street, S.E.
Grand Rapids, MI 49512
Tel: 800-626-1762
Fax: 616-942-1973

COUNTRY TECHNOLOGY, INC.
P.O. Box 87
Gays Mills, WI 54631
Tel: 608-735-4718
Fax: 608-735-4859

PARAGON SPORTING GOODS
867 Broadway
New York, NY 10003
Tel: 212-255-8036
Fax: 212-929-1831

CONTAINER FOR THE WEIGHTS

Always keep your dumbbells in a sturdy container or on a rack when you're not actually lifting them. Possibilities include a strong canvas tote bag or duffel bag (the handles are convenient) or a sturdy box.

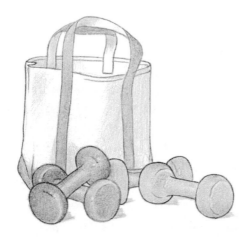

CHAIR

You'll do some of the exercises while seated in a chair, and for other moves you'll stand and hold the back of the chair for balance. Select a chair that's sturdy, with a seat high and deep enough so that when you sit back in it, your knee joint is just over the edge. To allow for free movement, the chair should be armless. Also, be sure the back is high enough so you can hold on to it without leaning over.

CLOTHING

You don't need special clothes for strength training—very handy if you do the exercises during a break at work. Clothing needs to be loose enough so you can move freely, and breathable so you don't get hot. Sneakers or athletic shoes are best; other low-heel shoes are acceptable, so long as they're flexible and sturdy.

WHAT ABOUT OTHER TYPES OF STRENGTH-TRAINING EQUIPMENT?

Women sometimes ask me about exercise elastic bands, because they're light and inexpensive. Though bands can be very beneficial, it's difficult to follow a progressive program with them, and they can be cumbersome to use correctly. Therefore, I prefer dumbbells.

Strength-training machines—both at-home and gym versions—can give you a terrific workout. To follow the *Strong Women Stay Slim* program with machines, just make sure you target the same muscle groups (the manual or a trainer can help). The same basic principles apply.

GENERAL INSTRUCTIONS FOR STRENGTH TRAINING

Strength training is safe for nearly everyone—especially if you heed the simple precautions below, which also make for more effective workouts.

CREATE A SAFE EXERCISE AREA

Clear a space for training that's large enough for your chair plus dumbbells. If possible, place the chair on a secure carpet, so it doesn't slide. If your floors are bare, stabilize the chair by putting it against a wall.

BACK SAFETY TIPS

Caution: if you've ever had back problems, or if you have osteoporosis, discuss this program with your doctor before you begin.

The following tips are for everyone—but pay special attention if you need to pamper your back:

◆ Be just as careful when moving weights to and from the workout area as you are when you do the exercises.

◆ If possible, store your dumbbells next to your workout area, so you don't have to move them for each session.

◆ Lift the container properly: bend at the legs and rise slowly.

Store your dumbbells in a container when you're not using them. As soon as you finish an exercise, put away the weights. Never leave dumbbells on a table or shelf—it's all too easy for them to roll off and drop on a foot. **Keep weights safely away from children and pets.**

◆　◆　◆

Even my 6-year-old niece has noticed that I'm strong. The other day she said to me: "Mommy can't pick me up anymore, but you can. I know why—it's because you lift weights."
—Susan

◆　◆　◆

Maintain Good Posture

Proper posture helps avoid muscle strain and injury when you strength train—but that's just one of its benefits. Standing tall is the fastest way to look pounds lighter and years younger. As your back and abdominal muscles get stronger, good posture becomes easier and easier.

Whether you're sitting or standing, your body should be relaxed but straight, as if someone had fastened a string to the top of your head and was pulling you up. Check yourself in a mirror, or ask a friend to check you.

Perform the Lifts Slowly

Most of us, unless we watch ourselves, tend to perform the lifts too quickly or to speed up as a session continues. For safety and for best results, it's important to do the exercises slowly. If you simply swing the weight or drop it, you could injure your back or shoulders. What's more, your muscles won't get trained if momentum or gravity does the work.

Count Out Loud While You Exercise

Counting aloud reminds you to move slowly. Also, it assures proper breathing—if you're counting you're not likely to hold your breath, a common mistake.

Good posture

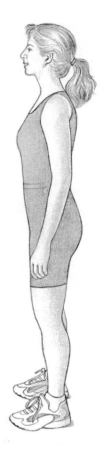

- ◆ Chin is tipped in, so it's in line with the neck.

- ◆ Neck is in line with the spine.

- ◆ Shoulders are back, down, and relaxed.

- ◆ Back is straight.

- ◆ Pelvis is slightly tucked under.

- ◆ Knees are not locked.

PROGRESS AT THE RECOMMENDED PACE

Some women become so enthusiastic about strength training that they press forward prematurely and attempt to lift weights that are too heavy. Try to be patient. If you advance too soon, you'll find it hard to maintain proper form and you could hurt yourself. Your tendons and ligaments, which generally aren't as strong as your muscles, need time to catch up. When you progress slowly, everything gets strong together.

It's important to allow at least one day for your muscles to recover between exercise sessions. Strength training creates microscopic tears in muscles, an accelerated version of the normal wear and tear from everyday life. What makes you stronger is the body's repair and rebuilding process, and that takes a little time.

RELAX!

In the instructions for each exercise, I'll remind you to check your body for tension—and to relax.

- **Face:** Keep your face relaxed; don't furrow or knit your brow.

- **Jaw and neck:** Avoid clenching your teeth or tightening your jaw. If your jaw is relaxed, your neck will be relaxed too.

- **Shoulders:** Don't scrunch your shoulders up toward your ears. Keep them back and relaxed.

- **Legs and arms:** Only the muscles you're exercising should be tensed. All other muscles in your body should be relaxed. Don't lock your knees.

If you need to stop strength training for two or more weeks, don't expect to resume at the point where you were before. Reduce the amount you lift, or drop back to an easier version of the exercises, just to be on the safe side; you can always increase the weight again as your muscles readjust.

◆ ◆ ◆

Every September there's a river cleanup day in my community. Last year I mainly watched. But this year I put waders on and pulled trash out of the water. Under a railroad bridge there were huge pieces of rails and old train switches. A group of men were there, waiting for other men to help them. I have prematurely white hair, so they probably thought I was someone's grandmother. I started hauling out these big pieces of rusted metal—30, 40, 50 pounds. They were very surprised.
  —Isabel

◆ ◆ ◆

SIX BASIC STRENGTH-TRAINING EXERCISES

The basic program calls for three twenty-minute exercise sessions per week; each session includes six exercises plus a stretch. It's a good idea to warm your muscles to prepare them for a workout. The first exercise in this program—the chair stand—serves as a warm-up.

In strength training, a complete move is called a **lift** or repetition. In this program, eight repetitions, or reps, make a **set**, and you do two sets of each exercise. A lift takes about nine seconds: four seconds to raise the weight, a one-second pause, and four seconds to return to the starting position. You'll stop for a few seconds to take a breath between lifts. Rest about one minute between sets. Though it's not necessary, you may want to pause for a minute or two when you finish an exercise before you go on to the next.

You'll start with light weights or the easiest version of the exercise. In the beginning you'll progress rapidly, and within a few weeks you'll be training at the proper intensity: you'll be able to perform each exercise eight times in good form, but this effort should be close to your limit. When the eighth lift is no longer a challenge, it's time to increase the load.

CHAIR STAND

This super exercise tackles several important muscle groups at once. You'll strengthen and tone your thighs, and work your back and abdominal muscles as well as your buttocks. Chair stands also improve your balance. Plus, this exercise is a great warm-up—which is why it comes first.

Start with Version 1. After that's no longer a challenge, move to Version 2, which is considerably more difficult. Some women can advance to Version 2 almost immediately. Others will find even Version 1 difficult. In that case, you can use your hands to help you rise and sit down again. And in a few weeks you should be able to do it without hands.

Version I

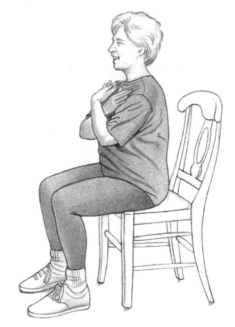

Starting position

Sit toward the front of the chair seat, with your feet flat on the floor, shoulder-width apart. Cross your arms and hold them against your chest, your left fingertips touching your right shoulder and your right fingertips touching your left shoulder.

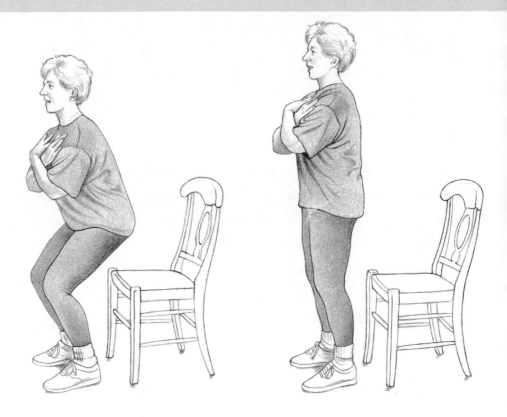

The move

◆ **1-2-3-Up:** Keeping your back straight, lean forward slightly and stand up *slowly*. The entire effort should come from your leg and buttock muscles.

◆ **Pause for a breath.**

◆ **1-2-3-Down:** *Slowly* return to the starting position. Do not let yourself fall into the chair!

◆ **Pause for a breath, then repeat.**

Where you will feel the effort

In your thighs and buttocks.

Sets and reps

Do eight repetitions for one set. Rest for a minute or two and do a second set.

Notes

The key to success with this exercise is to move slowly, especially as you return to the chair. Use your leg and buttock muscles to lower yourself—*don't* fall back into the seat. If this move is difficult, use your hands to make it easier.

- Remember to move slowly.
- Lean just slightly forward as you start the move.
- Don't hold your breath.
- Check for tension, and relax.

Version 2: Reverse Chair Stand

This version increases effort in two ways: first, it adds the weight of your outstretched arms; second, it's based on a standing rather than seated position. As a result, your abdominal and lower back muscles have to work harder. Don't attempt to do the Reverse Chair Stand until

▼ ▼ ▼ ▼ ▼ ▼ ▼ ▼ ▼ ▼ ▼ ▼ ▼ ▼ ▼ ▼

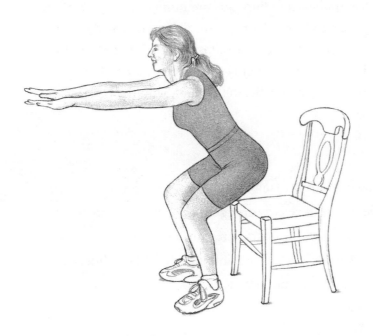

Version 1 has become easy for you. Later you can make Version 2 even tougher by lowering yourself almost to the chair, but not actually touching it before you pause and rise again.

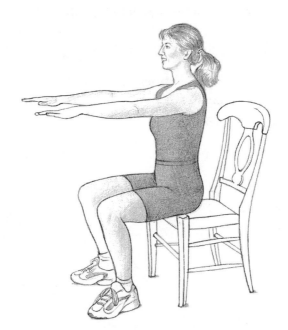

Starting position

Sit down in the chair, then stand up; this preliminary move assures that you're a safe distance from the chair and won't land on the floor when you sit during the exercise. Stand in front of the chair with head high, feet shoulder-width apart, toes slightly turned out. Extend both arms straight out in front of you, parallel to the floor, with the palms facing down.

The move

◆ **1-2-3-Sit:** Slowly lower yourself into the chair. Keep your chin up, with your eyes facing forward throughout the move. Bend at your hips, keeping your back straight. Aim your buttocks backward and lean forward. *Don't* let yourself fall into the chair! The effort should come from your muscles, not gravity.

◆ **Pause for a breath.**

◆ **1-2-3-Stand:** Slowly raise yourself back to the starting position.

◆ **Pause for a breath, then repeat.**

Where you will feel the effort

In your thighs, buttocks, and trunk.

Sets and reps

Do eight repetitions for one set. Rest for a minute or two and do a second set.

Notes

- Remember to move slowly.
- Don't bend so far forward that your knees move in front of your toes; knees should remain above your ankles.
- Don't hold your breath.
- Check for tension, and relax.

◆ ◆ ◆

I once got stuck on a low sofa at a friend's house, and it was so embarrassing—I had to ask her to pull me up. This would never happen now that I've lost weight and strengthened my legs.
—Alexandra

◆ ◆ ◆

OVERHEAD PRESS

Here's a great exercise for your arms and shoulders. The muscles of the shoulders and the backs of the upper arms are notoriously weak in women. That's why it's so difficult to hoist heavy objects over your head—as you may have discovered if you've ever tried to lift a suitcase into the overhead compartment on an airplane. Toning these muscles firms those unwelcome "batwings" on the backs of upper arms, and contributes to good posture. Another bonus: improved flexibility. Suddenly you can reach that back zipper!

Starting position

Stand straight with a dumbbell in each hand, feet shoulder-width (about sixteen to eighteen inches) apart. Hold the dumbbells up, parallel to the floor, with the inner ends touching the front sides of your shoulders. Your palms should face forward.

The move

◆ **1-2-3-Up:** Push the dumbbells straight up from the starting position until your arms are over your head. The dumbbells should be slightly in front of your body when your arms are fully extended.

◆ **Pause for a breath.**

◆ **1-2-3-Down:** Slowly lower the dumbbells back to the starting position.

◆ **Pause for a breath, then repeat.**

Where you will feel the effort

In your upper arms, shoulders, and upper back.

Sets and reps

Do eight repetitions for one set. Rest for a minute or two and do a second set.

Notes

◆ Make sure the dumbbells don't move forward or out to the side as you perform the lift; they should go straight up.

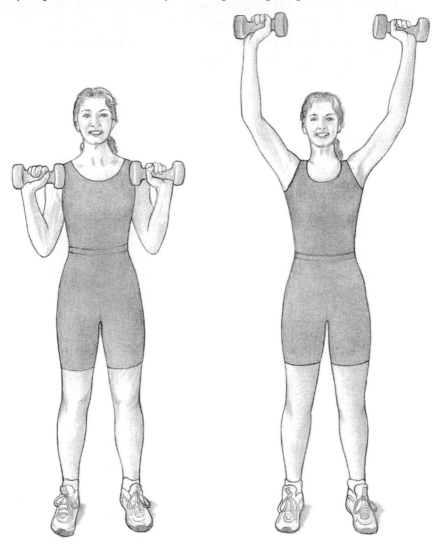

- Maintain good posture; don't scrunch your shoulders or arch your back.

- Move slowly.

- Don't hold your breath.

- Check for tension, and relax.

◆ ◆ ◆

I like the fact that I'm building muscle—it makes me feel like a fuel-burning engine. I like feeling stronger. I think it's really important for women to get strong. You don't feel as dependent; you don't always have to ask your husband for help.
—Jane

◆ ◆ ◆

BENT-OVER ROW

Several important muscle groups get a workout from this exercise. You'll train the biceps muscles in front of your upper arms, as well as back and shoulder muscles. Your back and abdominal muscles are challenged too, since they work hard to keep your torso stable. Don't be surprised if people start asking if you've lost weight—as your upper body gets stronger, you'll automatically stand taller, which makes you look slimmer.

Starting position

Sit forward in the chair with your feet flat on the floor, shoulder-width (sixteen to eighteen inches) apart, with a dumbbell in each hand. Let your arms hang down at your sides, palms facing in. Contract your ab-

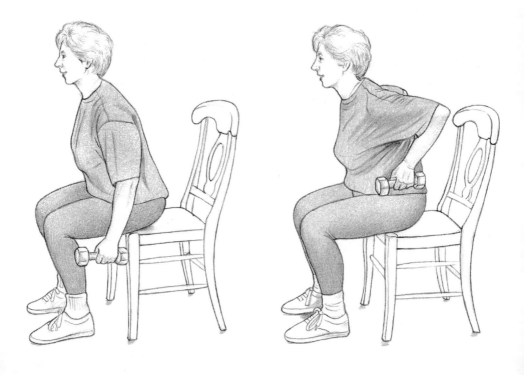

dominal muscles to hold your torso stable—this will help firm your abs. Bend slightly forward at the waist, with your back straight, until your chest is just above your thighs. Your arms will move forward slightly until they're just behind your lower legs, parallel to them.

The move

◆ **1-2-3-Up:** Using your shoulder and upper back muscles, pull both dumbbells straight up as high as you can. Your shoulder blades should move closer together. Your elbows will need to bend, but most of the effort should come from your shoulders and back. Keep your wrists straight during the move. At the top of the lift, your elbows should point back—or as close to that direction as you can manage.

◆ **Pause for a breath.**

◆ **1-2-3-Down:** Slowly lower the dumbbells to the starting position.

◆ **Pause for a breath, then repeat.**

Where you will feel the effort

In your upper back, upper arms, and shoulders, as well as your lower back and abdomen; in your thighs, because these muscles work to hold your body stable while you do the exercise.

Sets and reps

Do eight repetitions for one set. Rest for a minute or two and do a second set.

Notes

Caution: if you have osteoporosis, talk with your doctor before you do this exercise.

▼   ▼   ▼   ▼   ▼   ▼   ▼   ▼   ▼   ▼   ▼   ▼   ▼   ▼   ▼   ▼   ▼   ▼   ▼

In the beginning, your elbows may point to the sides. As you become slimmer, stronger, and more flexible, you'll be able to point your elbows farther back. Similarly, if your abdomen is large, you might have trouble leaning forward. Just bend as far as is comfortable and perform the lift.

- Make sure your head, neck, and back are in a straight line. Don't flex or arch your back.
- Though you're supposed to bring your shoulder blades together, don't scrunch your shoulders up toward your ears.
- Move slowly.
- Don't hold your breath.
- Check for tension, and relax.

CALF RAISE

Toned calf muscles give curves as well as strength to your lower legs. This exercise also strengthens your ankle joints and makes them more flexible. These changes improve your balance and add power to every move you make on your feet, whether it's walking, climbing stairs, or cross-country skiing.

As your calves get stronger and your balance improves, try to perform this exercise with less assistance from your hands. Eventually, you may be able to do it with hands poised above the chair but not holding on.

Starting position

Stand behind a sturdy chair that has a back high enough for you to hold for balance. Stand with feet shoulder-width apart, fingertips resting lightly on the back of the chair.

The move

- **1-2-3-Up:** Slowly raise yourself up as high as you can on the balls of your feet.
- **Hold for three seconds.**
- **1-2-3-Down:** Slowly lower your heels back to the starting position.
- **Pause for a breath, then repeat.**

Where you will feel the effort

In your ankles, feet, and calves.

Sets and reps

Do eight repetitions for one set. Rest for a minute or two and do a second set.

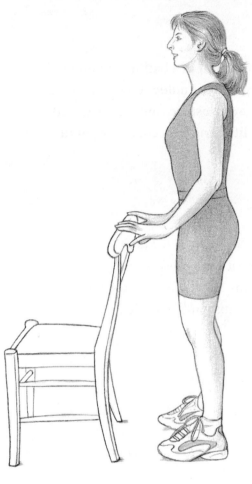

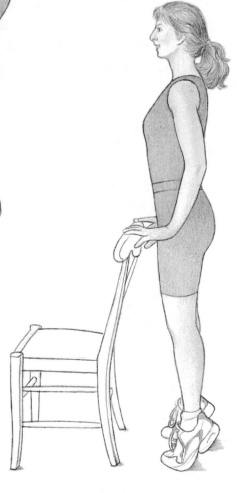

Notes

- ◆ Check your posture; make sure you stand up straight.
- ◆ Move slowly.
- ◆ Don't hold your breath.
- ◆ Check for tension, and relax—make sure your knee joints are relaxed, not locked or hyperextended.

SEATED FLY

Strong, shapely shoulders look beautiful in a bathing suit or tank top. This exercise really concentrates on the shoulder muscles. Stronger shoulder muscles contribute to good posture, and they help with heavy lifting. The move can be a little tricky to coordinate at first, but it's easy once you learn it.

Starting position

Sit forward in the chair with your feet flat on the floor shoulder-width apart. With your upper arms against your sides, grasp one dumbbell in each hand, palms facing your thighs. Bend your elbows slightly. Your hands will be just in front of your hips, on the outside of your thighs.

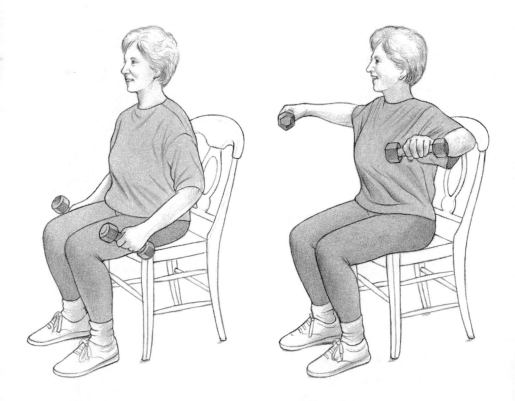

▼ ▼ ▼ ▼ ▼ ▼ ▼ ▼ ▼ ▼ ▼ ▼ ▼ ▼ ▼ ▼ ▼ ▼

The move

- **1-2-3-Up:** Slowly lift your upper arms straight out to the sides, maintaining the same slight bend in your elbow. At the end of the lift, your upper arms will be parallel to the floor and straight out to the sides of your shoulders. Your forearms, still slightly bent, will also be parallel to the floor.
- **Pause for a breath.**
- **1-2-3-Down:** In a smooth motion, lower your arms back to the starting position.
- **Pause for a breath, then repeat.**

Where you will feel the effort

In your shoulders and upper arms.

Sets and reps

Do eight repetitions for one set. Rest for a minute or two and do a second set.

Notes

This exercise can be confusing at first, but the move is very fluid and easy once you learn it. Most women need to use a lighter dumbbell for this exercise than for the others, because this muscle is usually weaker.

- Throughout the move, keep your elbow just slightly bent. The effort should come from your shoulder muscles.
- Don't scrunch your shoulders.
- Don't let your arms come above shoulder height.
- Move slowly.
- Don't hold your breath.
- Check for tension, and relax.

ARM CURL

Women love this exercise—which strengthens the biceps—because it gets fast results. You'll feel the difference when you're lifting grocery bags or acing a tennis serve. And your arms will look great too.

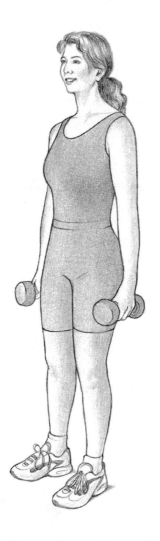
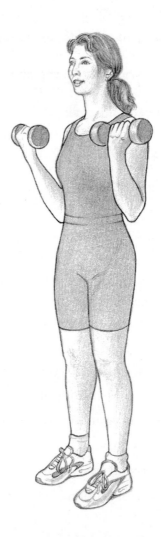

Starting position

Stand with your feet shoulder-width apart, with your arms down at your sides holding the dumbbells. Palms should face in, toward your legs.

The move

◆ **1-2-3-Up:** Keeping your elbows gently pressed against your sides, raise the dumbbells by bringing your forearms up. The dumbbells should move from your sides to the front of your shoulders in one smooth motion. Your elbows will bend; your forearms will rotate; and your wrists will remain straight. At the end of the move, the dumbbells will be at shoulder height, parallel to the floor, with your palms facing your shoulders.

◆ **Pause for a breath.**

◆ **1-2-3-Down:** Lower your arms, smoothly rotating your forearms so the dumbbells return to the starting position, with palms facing in. Keep your elbows gently anchored at your sides through the entire movement.

◆ **Pause for a breath, then repeat.**

Where you will feel the effort

In your upper arms.

Sets and reps

Do eight repetitions for one set. Rest for a minute or two and do a second set.

Notes

◆ Maintain good posture; don't arch your back.

◆ Don't bend your wrists.

◆ Keep your elbows anchored at your sides.

◆ Move slowly.

◆ Don't hold your breath.

◆ Check for tension, a

STRETCH

A brief stretch after a strength-training session helps prevent injury
and contributes to flexibility. If you're doing aerobic exercise and
strength training in the same workout, begin with aerobics to warm
your muscles, then strength train—and save the stretching for the end.
It's a wonderful way to relax after vigorous exercise.

The basic instructions for stretching are very simple: get into the
position, extending your muscles as far as you comfortably can. Hold
the stretch for twenty to thirty seconds,
breathing normally. During the stretch,
gently try to extend the position, but never
go to the point of discomfort. Try to relax
your muscles as much as possible—the
more you relax, the more your muscles will
be able to stretch.

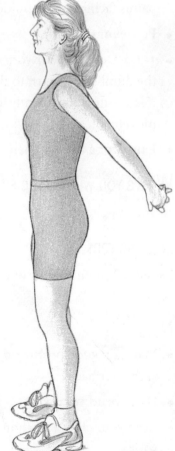

Shoulder Stretch

This move stretches the muscles of
your shoulders and upper arms.
Stand with your feet shoulder-
width apart, arms at your sides.
Extend your arms straight behind
your body, pulling them back and
up as high as you can. You may
clasp your hands together, if you're
able to do so.

Quadriceps Stretch

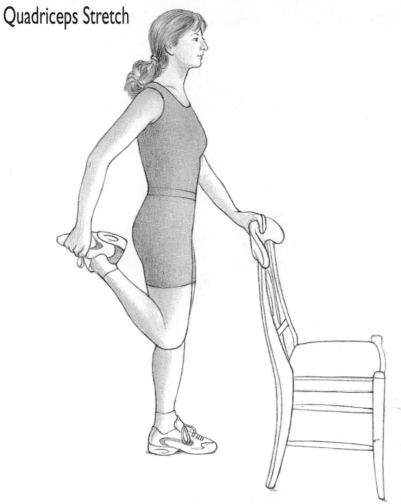

Stand next to the chair. Holding on with your left hand, bend your right knee so your right leg comes up behind you. Grasp your ankle and hold it, pointing your knee down (or as close to down as possible). Hold the stretch for twenty to thirty seconds, then release. Repeat, switching so that you hold on to the chair with your right hand and bend your left knee.

Note: at first, you may not be able to reach your ankle when you bend your knee and raise your leg behind you. In that case, just bend your knee and bring your lower leg back; keep your thigh perpendicular to the ground and your lower leg parallel to the floor.

Lower Back and Hamstring Stretch

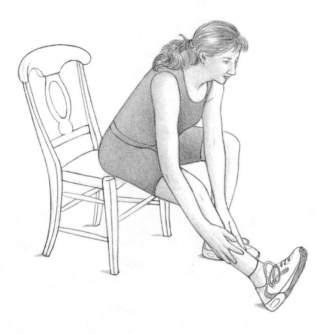

Sit forward in a chair with your feet flat on the floor. Your thighs and lower legs should form a right angle. Slide your right leg forward, keeping your heel on the floor, until your right knee is straight, but not locked. Your ankle should be relaxed. Extend both arms, pointing your fingers toward your right foot. Bend as far toward your right foot as you comfortably can. Hold the stretch for twenty seconds, then release. Repeat, this time extending your left leg.

Lower Leg and Ankle Stretch

Sit in a chair with your feet flat on the floor. Extend your legs slightly so that your heels are one to two inches off the floor. Flex your toes up and bend your ankles back toward you as much as you can. Hold the stretch for twenty to thirty seconds, then point your toes down and bend your feet away from you as far as possible. Hold the stretch for twenty to thirty seconds.

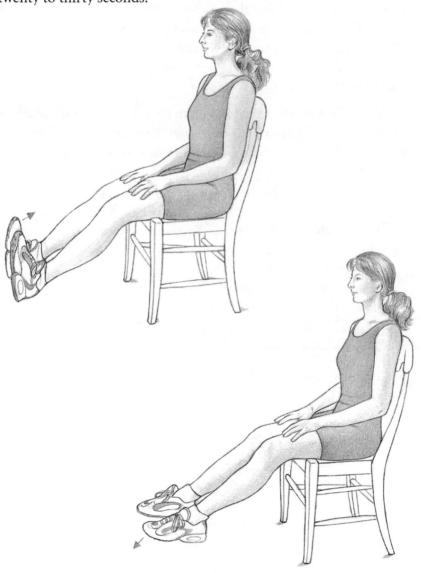

CREATING AN INDIVIDUALIZED PROGRAM

You've learned the moves. The next step is to turn the exercises into an *individualized program* that will increase your strength. This program will be simple—but not easy! To get strong, you must train at a challenging level. As you become stronger, you'll need to adjust to maintain that challenge. Using the right weights or version for each exercise is the key to both safety and success. If you overdo it, you'll find the program unnecessarily difficult. On the other hand, if you expect too little of yourself, you won't see the kind of progress that makes strength training so exciting.

Where to Start

The greatest amount of weight you can lift just once is your maximum strength capacity. You'll be working out at 70 to 80 percent of your maximum. This means the lifts are well within your ability, yet the effort is great enough to improve your strength. For safety's sake, you'll start at a level that's considerably lower—no more than 50 to 60 percent—while you're learning the moves.

- If you're already following the *Strong Women Stay Young* program or another strength-training program, but you want to switch to the exercises in this book, start with weights that are the same or lower than what you're using now. For a familiar exercise, use your customary weight; if the exercise is new, use your lightest weight and increase after a session or two.

- If you've never strength trained before (or haven't done so recently) and are in good health, start with 1-pound weights.

- If you have health concerns, discuss the program with your doctor before you start. One option to consider is beginning the exercises without weights.

Your first few sessions probably will seem a little too easy, but in my experience that's helpful when you're mastering proper form. Within a few weeks, you'll reach the right intensity. After that, you'll add weight or move to the next version as your muscles strengthen. The program will always be right for your body.

How to Evaluate Your Effort

The scale on the next page—inspired by the Borg Exercise Intensity Scale that many researchers use—will help you recognize when you're working out at the right intensity.

The right effort for strength training is Level 4. You should find the weight moderately difficult to lift the first time, but well within your capability. By the third or fourth lift, it should seem heavier. Ideally you should be able to perform the eighth lift in good form, but feel that if you didn't stop and rest your muscles, you couldn't continue.

Working out at Level 3 (except for the first few weeks) is not sufficiently challenging; it will increase your endurance, but not your strength. On the other hand, training at Level 5 is risky—if the effort is too great, you won't be able to maintain proper form and you might injure yourself.

With the chair stand, which uses body weight, you won't be able to adjust your effort quite so precisely. Aim to move to the next higher version as soon as you can do so without exceeding Level 4 intensity. If you aren't sure, wait. It's better to progress more slowly than to work your muscles too hard.

Finding the Right Challenge

I've given you a very conservative starting point—just 1 pound in most cases—so you can focus on your form, on breathing and relaxing, and on establishing the slow rhythm of lifting and lowering a weight. By the fourth week you should be training at Level 4 intensity.

Week 1:

Stay at the starting level for all three sessions to learn the exercises, even if it's too easy. If your first session seems too hard, or if your muscles are very uncomfortable afterward, do the exercises without weights.

Week 2:

For the exercises that use dumbbells, add up to 1 pound per session, as needed to increase effort to Level 4. However, if your muscles are sore, con-

EXERCISE INTENSITY SCALE for STRENGTH TRAINING	
LEVEL	DESCRIPTION OF EFFORT
1	Very easy: too easy to be noticed; like lifting a pencil.
2	Easy: can be felt, but isn't fatiguing; like carrying a book.
3	Moderate: fatiguing only if prolonged; like carrying a full handbag that seems heavier as the day goes on.
4	Hard: more than moderate at first, and becoming difficult by the time you complete six or seven repetitions. You can make the effort eight times in good form, but need to rest afterward.
5	Extremely hard: requires all your strength, like lifting a piece of heavy furniture that you can only lift once, if at all.

tinue with the same weight or, if the discomfort is bothersome, decrease the weight. You may find that you need to add weights on some exercises but not others. That's normal, because the strength of different muscles varies.

Week 3:

Aim to be working out at Level 4 on all the exercises by the end of this week. (You'll also begin your aerobics program this week—more about that in Chapter 8.) Don't be surprised if you're using different dumbbells for different exercises.

Working Toward Goals

After the initial adjustment, try to increase the weight for each exercise every week. Of course, you shouldn't attempt to work out at Level 5. But you'll make more progress if you push yourself to stay at the top of the Level 4 range rather than waiting so long to increase the weight that your effort has dropped to Level 3.

Sometimes you'll find yourself between dumbbells or versions—what you're doing seems too easy, but the next step up is too difficult. The best way to make the transition is to use your current weight or version for the first set, then move up for the second set. After a few sessions, you'll be ready to do both sets in good form at the more challenging intensity.

Weekly changes won't always be possible. Also, you'll soon see that progress is easier with some exercises than with others. The wide range of individual responses always fascinates me. Some women move forward rapidly;

STRENGTH-TRAINING GOALS			
Exercise	20 to 49 years old	50 to 69 years old	70 years and older
Chair stand	Version 2	Version 2	Version 2
Overhead press	12–15 pounds	10–12 pounds	8–10 pounds
Bent-over row	12–15 pounds	10–12 pounds	8–10 pounds
Calf raise	No hands, if possible	No hands, if possible	No hands, if possible
Seated fly	8–10 pounds	5–8 pounds	5–8 pounds
Arm curl	12–15 pounds	10–12 pounds	8–10 pounds

others advance more slowly. There are certain common patterns, though. Most people find the arm curl considerably easier than the seated fly and overhead press. That's because the arm curl uses the biceps muscles, which tend to be a lot stronger than the triceps in the back of the arm (used for the overhead press) and the shoulder muscles (used for the seated fly). Don't be discouraged—all of your muscle groups will become stronger.

The preceding table shows strength goals by age and exercise. When you're training at these levels, you will have obtained most of the health benefits you can expect from a strengthening program—provided you keep it up. Most women reach these goals after six to nine months on this program, or at least come close.

These goals are by no means upper limits. Studies that follow people for as long as two years find that they keep improving, though of course the changes become very slow. How much further you go is up to you. My personal preference is to maintain healthy levels, rather than struggling to surpass them.

WHEN YOU'RE READY FOR MORE

I've included two optional extra exercises to further strengthen the muscles of your back and abdomen, as well as your lower body. All use your own weight for resistance. I encourage you to include them in your program, but not right away. You'll have a lot to learn when you start the *Strong Women Stay Slim* program—the basic strengthening exercises, plus your aerobics exercises and the food plan. That's plenty for the first four weeks. After that, you can add the extra moves if you wish. Perform the new moves right after the chair stands, then continue with the other five exercises of the basic six, and end with your stretches.

PELVIC TILT

This exercise is a classic—and for good reason. One simple move firms and strengthens your entire midsection: buttocks, thighs, abdomen, and back. It's a perfect complement to the basic program. You can do the exercise on a firm mattress or padded bench if you'd rather not get down on the floor.

Starting position

Lie on your back with your knees bent and feet flat on the floor, shoulder-width apart. Your arms should be at your sides and relaxed, with palms flat.

The move

◆ **1-2-3-Up:** Slowly roll your pelvis off the floor—first your hips, then your waist, and finally your lower back. Your midsection should form a straight line from your knees to your upper back. Your shoulders will remain on the floor.

◆ **Pause for a breath.**

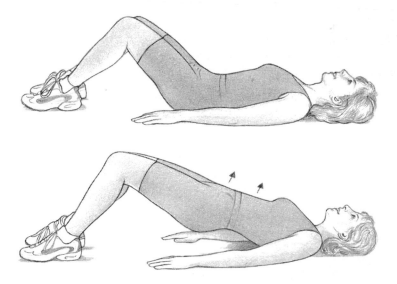

- **1-2-3-Down:** Slowly roll back to the starting position, lowering first your back, then your waist, and finally your hips.

- **Pause for a breath, then repeat.**

Where you will feel the effort

In the front and back of your thighs, buttocks, abdomen, and lower back.

Sets and reps

Do eight repetitions for one set. Rest briefly and do another set of eight repetitions.

Notes

Caution: this exercise puts pressure on your upper back. If you have osteoporosis or back problems, check with your doctor before trying it.

- If you find the move uncomfortable, don't roll quite as far back.

- When you lower yourself, your movement should be controlled; don't drop onto the floor.

- Move smoothly and slowly.

- Don't hold your breath.

- Check for tension, and relax.

FRONT LEG RAISE

Here's an excellent thigh-shaper. The bonus is added leg strength, which helps when you're walking, playing sports, or rising from a chair.

Starting position

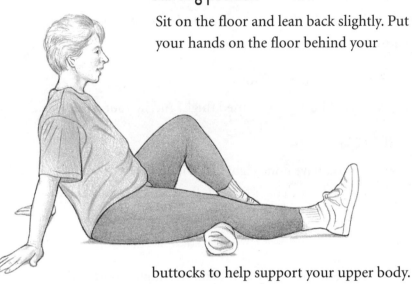

Sit on the floor and lean back slightly. Put your hands on the floor behind your

buttocks to help support your upper body. Extend your legs straight in front of you. Put a rolled-up towel under your right knee to keep you from locking your knee. Your left knee should be bent, with your left foot on the floor next to your right leg, just above the ankle.

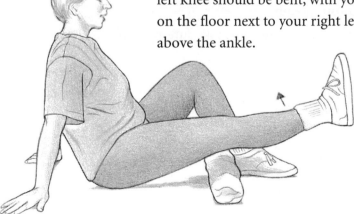

The move

◆ **1-2-3-Up:** Slowly lift your right leg as high as possible—this may be as little as four inches in the beginning, up to sixteen inches when you become stronger and more flexible. Keep your right leg straight with the foot relaxed and toes pointing up.

◆ **Pause for a breath.**

◆ **1-2-3-Down:** Slowly lower your right leg to the floor.

◆ **Pause for a breath, then repeat.**

Where you will feel the effort

In the front and back of the raised thigh, and in your lower back.

Sets and reps

Repeat until you have done eight lifts with your right leg; then do eight lifts with your left leg. That's one set. Rest for a minute or two, then do a second set.

Notes

As you become stronger, try to lift your leg higher off the floor.

◆ The movement should be slow and controlled; don't let your leg drop.

◆ Don't round your back or slump your shoulders.

◆ Don't hold your breath.

◆ Check for tension, and relax—make sure your toes are relaxed.

To Readers of
Strong Women Stay Young

I f you've been following the program in my first book, *Strong Women Stay Young (SWSY)*, you may be puzzled to see that the exercises in this book are different, and that I recommend three strength-training sessions per week instead of two.

The *Strong Women Stay Slim* program calls for three strength-training sessions per week because it's designed for weight loss—an extra session revs up your metabolism even more and helps preserve muscle and bone as you lose weight. Because you're doing three sessions and also aerobic exercise, I streamlined the strength training. That's why I didn't include exercises with ankle weights.

If you've been following the program in *SWSY* and want to continue, by all means do so. But if you're losing weight, consider doing three *SWSY* sessions per week instead of two. If you'd like to combine the two programs, here are some guidelines so you don't overwork the same muscles:

- **Arm exercises:** Do the biceps curls following either *SWSY* or this book. Do either the overhead triceps from *SWSY* or the overhead press from this book. And do all the other arm exercises—the bent-over row and seated fly from this book, and the upward row from *SWSY*. If you want to omit one of these three, drop the upward row.

- **Leg exercises:** If you want to continue working out with ankle weights, stick with the leg exercises in *SWSY*. You can add the chair stands from this book if you wish—indeed, I suggested using them for a warm-up in *SWSY*. If you prefer not to use the ankle weights, just do the chair stands and the calf raises from this book; add the heel stands from *SWSY* if you wish.

EASE YOURSELF

INTO FITNESS

*When I'm under stress and my shoulders are up around my ears,
I go for a swim or a run. It gets all the tension out. My energy level
is much higher; I feel much better; my back doesn't hurt. I'm fitting into things again. I had been size 14 going on 16. Now I'm almost in size 12.*

　　—Nancy

◆　　◆　　◆

A erobic activity is one of the great health tonics—and a terrific calorie
burner. Once your body is strong and fit, it's a joy to be physically active.

I realize that you may be unaccustomed to aerobic exercise. If so, you
can start slowly. Indeed, you don't have to begin the aerobic portion of the
Strong Women Stay Slim program until the third week, and your first session
can be as brief as ten minutes. From this modest beginning, you'll steadily
progress until, by the tenth week, you will have reached the standard for vigorous physical activity suggested by the American College of Sports Medicine, the U.S. Surgeon General, and the U.S. Centers for Disease Control and
Prevention. This is no small feat: according to recent surveys, at least three-
quarters of American women don't meet the recommended minimum. In ad-

dition, I expect you'll feel more energetic and be more active throughout the day, which is important for weight loss too.

AEROBIC OPTIONS

I think it's helpful to have one "daily bread" exercise—something you can count on doing three to six times a week, which easily becomes a routine part of your life. Any sustained activity that elevates your heart rate is acceptable for this program.

If you're already doing exercise of this kind, that's great! Just continue, adjusting as necessary to progress toward the fitness goals described later in the chapter. If you've been sedentary, I suggest you select one aerobic activity for the first few weeks. Once you become familiar with it, you can expand your repertoire. Variety will prevent boredom; also, different activities strengthen different muscles.

Women often ask me, "What's the best aerobic activity?" My answer: **The best activity is one you enjoy and that's easy for you to do regularly**.

My mother, who's 70 years old and lives in Vermont, cross-country skis five days a week during the winter and mountain bikes in the summer. Cross-country skiing is my favorite way to exercise, but unlike my mom, I can't do it frequently. Because I've been a competitive athlete I need a strenuous activity to maintain my fitness level, so my "daily bread" exercise is running. I run (or do something equally demanding) three to five times a week. In addition, I'm physically active every day—climbing stairs, walking, playing with my kids.

For many women, brisk walking is the ideal aerobic activity because it fits so easily into their lives. But if you don't enjoy walking, or find it painful or impractical, it's not the best exercise for you. Fortunately, there are many other options.

♦ ♦ ♦

I live in a hot climate with a long summer, and a swim before dinner revives me. I swim various strokes to make sure I'm training all my muscles. It's a wonderful spirit-lifter. Sometimes I think out

*a problem while I'm doing laps. Other times I don't think at all.
Even though it's hard work, when I'm finished I always feel re-
laxed, as if the worries of the day have dissolved in the water.*
 —*Barbara*

◆ ◆ ◆

*My husband and I want our children to be active, and we've made
a commitment to be active as a family. We all took figure skating
lessons together. We go roller blading and horseback riding. We
really enjoy our adventures. The more active we are, the younger I
feel.*
 —*Isabel*

◆ ◆ ◆

*I use cardiovascular machines—mainly a treadmill and a recum-
bent stair climber—at a health club. I like the detailed feedback I
get from machines, because I can see even tiny progress, and that's
very encouraging. Also, I like working out at a gym: it's air-condi-
tioned, it's safe, and there's a bathroom nearby.*
 —*Sarah*

◆ ◆ ◆

GENERAL INSTRUCTIONS

A few basic measures will make your aerobic workouts more effective, safer, and much more enjoyable.

DRESS FOR SUCCESS

Comfortable clothes keep your workout pleasurable, and even protect you. Some women get a boost from stylish exercise gear, but if you prefer to keep it simple, a loose cotton T-shirt and shorts or leggings are just fine.

- ◆ Dress for the weather. On cold days, wear layers that you can peel off as your body warms up. When it's warm, wear light colors outdoors (dark colors absorb heat from the sun). Select cotton garments or look for new materials that help draw sweat away from your skin.

◆ Dress for safety. If you're working out on equipment, wear clothing that can't get caught in moving parts. Use all recommended safety gear, such as a helmet if you're biking, or reflecting strips on clothing if you walk at night.

◆ Protect yourself from the sun if you exercise outdoors. Wear sunscreen and sunglasses, plus a hat with a visor.

◆ Wear a supportive, comfortable brassiere that allows free movement.

◆ Wear clean socks made from an absorbent material. Make sure they fit well, with no folds or seams that chafe your feet. Keep your toenails clipped so they don't push up against another toe or the end of your shoe.

◆ Select shoes that fit well and that are appropriate for your activity. Good athletic shoes can be expensive, but they're worth it because they help prevent injuries and discomfort. Note: if your shoes are a year old, chances are they need replacement or repair. Examine footwear at least once a month. When you become active, you'll find that shoes wear out more quickly.

Select Safe Surroundings

If you exercise outdoors, take sensible precautions. Avoid unsafe neighborhoods and dangerous traffic. If the weather is bad, watch for slippery surfaces when you're biking, running, or walking. Try to find an exercise buddy (or at least stick to well-populated routes), especially at night.

Check the Equipment

If you're using equipment—bicycle, stationary cycle, treadmill, etc.—give it a quick look-over before each workout to make sure it's in good repair. Follow all maintenance suggestions in the manual.

CAUTION

Remember to take the Par-Q (see page 98) before you begin this or any other exercise program.

If you follow the instructions in this book, it's extremely unlikely that you'll ever experience any of the symptoms below. But if you do, use common sense: stop training immediately. And if the symptom persists, contact your medical caregiver.

◆ Chest pain or pressure

◆ Dizziness or light-headedness

◆ Nausea

◆ Sweating not explained by physical effort or by hot flashes

◆ Any unusual or worsening pain—for instance, pain in a joint; or pain in the jaw or in the arm or shoulder that's not caused by muscle fatigue

DRINK PLENTY OF WATER

During aerobic activity, your body requires extra water. You're evaporating water, in the form of perspiration, to keep cool. You're also releasing additional moisture through respiration, because you're breathing more rapidly. And your stepped-up metabolism is creating waste products that need to be flushed away. Consequently, for top performance during aerobic exercise, your body needs to be well hydrated.

To ensure you're getting enough, drink at least one cup of water during the hour before your workout. Then drink another cup or two within the forty-five minutes following aerobic activity. If an activity is prolonged—for instance, if you're taking a long hike or spending an afternoon gardening—drink a cup of water every hour or so. Your need for water will be even greater on hot days, when your body has to work harder to stay cool.

A simple way to monitor hydration is by glancing at your urine when you use the bathroom. Ideally, urine should be very pale yellow, almost clear. If it's dark, you're probably dehydrated.

LIMIT DISTRACTIONS

Exercise can be more enjoyable if you're listening to music or conversing with a friend. Some women like to read or watch TV while they ride their stationary cycle. That's fine, so long as the distraction doesn't interfere with a safe and effective workout. However, I don't recommend it at the beginning, when you're learning to use the equipment.

Two cautions if you wear headphones to listen to a personal stereo: first, keep the volume low enough to be kind to your ears. Second, if you're outdoors, make sure you can hear what's happening around you.

WARM UP

Muscles work best when they're warm: they're more elastic and have a better supply of blood. So it's important to warm your muscles before you place heavy demands on them. This is especially true for older people and those with cardiovascular disease.

A warm-up need not be elaborate. Just begin your exercise at a slow, easy pace, rather than at full speed. Take five minutes to reach your target intensity. This gradual transition from a resting to an active state gives your body time to adjust.

COOL DOWN AND STRETCH

After aerobic exercise, it's tempting to fall into a chair or to tear off your sweaty clothes and stand under the shower. Not yet! Your body needs to cool down first, and your muscles need a stretch.

When you're exercising at the proper intensity, your heart is pumping, your blood vessels are dilated, and your muscles are contracting to push blood back from your extremities to your heart. If you stop too abruptly, your heart is still pumping blood out, but your muscles are not returning it. This could make you feel dizzy or faint; in rare cases it could even cause serious heart irregularities. The problem can be exacerbated by heat, which is why a gradual cool-down is especially important if you plan to visit the sauna or steam room after exercising.

The cool-down is just as simple as the warm-up, only in reverse: over a five-minute period, slow your pace to the equivalent of a slow walk. Afterward you can do your strengthening exercises if you're combining the two into a single workout session.

End your exercise session with a stretch. Stretching is particularly important after an aerobic workout because most aerobic activities work your muscles at high intensity, but through only a limited range of motion. If you don't stretch afterward, you can actually decrease your flexibility. The four simple stretches described on pages 134–137 in Chapter 7 prevent that problem—and they feel great!

HOW TO GAUGE AEROBIC EFFORT

The key to getting results from aerobic exercise, just as with strength training, is to work out at the right intensity. When you do strength training, you use a weight you can lift eight times in good form—but no more—before you have to rest. You'll be aiming for a similar kind of challenge when you do aerobic exercise, but you'll use different indicators, including your heart rate.

When you do aerobic exercise in this program, your heart will work at about 60 to 70 percent of its maximum most of the time. This is safely within your capability, but high enough to give your cardiovascular system a good workout. How do you know you're at the right level? In the laboratory, we use heart-rate monitoring and a twenty-point exercise-intensity scale to measure aerobic effort. But in most cases, you can get all the information you need by referring to a very simple intensity scale or by checking your pulse.

ESTIMATING EXERCISE INTENSITY

The easiest way to measure aerobic effort is with a subjective scale that describes how you're feeling as you exercise. You can use the scale at any point in your workout, and you don't need special apparatus. Though this system generally works well, I encourage you also to take your pulse a few times (I'll tell you how in a minute), to make sure your impressions match your actual heart rate.

The *Strong Women Stay Slim* aerobics program calls for Level 3 effort. But I hope you'll also do considerably more Level 2 activity as you become stronger and more fit. The more active you are, the more calories and fat you

EXERCISE INTENSITY SCALE
FOR AEROBIC ACTIVITY

LEVEL	DESCRIPTION OF EFFORT
1—Sedentary	No perceived effort; standing, sitting, or lying down.
2—Active This level contributes to overall health and burns more calories than being sedentary.	Easy, sustainable movement that causes a small increase in heart and breathing rate and doesn't raise a sweat (unless the weather is hot); strolling, gardening, slow dancing, golfing.
3—Aerobic training You should exercise at this level to condition your heart and lungs.	Somewhat hard movement that elevates the heart rate to 60 to 70 percent of maximum most of the time, ranging up to 80 percent. Breathing is more rapid, though it's possible to converse with only slightly altered speech; perspiration appears after about five to fifteen minutes, depending on air temperature.
4—Athletic training This is a more advanced level of aerobic conditioning that might become an appropriate goal after the ten-week program.	Hard effort that elevates the heart rate to 70 to 80 percent most of the time, ranging up to 90 percent of maximum. Breathing is rapid but not labored—it's possible to converse, though faster breathing causes interruptions; perspiration starts within five to ten minutes, depending on air temperature; fatigue increases as the workout continues.
5—Over-exertion Not recommended!	Excessive effort: heart pounds to the point of discomfort or nausea; breathing is too rapid to permit speech.

burn. Indeed, **if you simply add half an hour of Level 2 activity a day for a year, without making any changes in your diet, you'll lose about ten pounds.**

Once you're familiar with the intensity scale, it will help you stay in touch with your body during your workouts. That's very important, because you'll need to adjust your exercise sessions over time. As you become fitter, you'll increase your pace to maintain the right level of challenge. If you catch a cold or miss sleep and feel temporarily run-down, you'll need to slow down for a day or more. These adjustments are easy and natural if you've learned how to listen to your body.

MEASURING YOUR HEART RATE

Heart-rate monitors can be purchased at sporting goods stores, but the good monitors are expensive (around $200). Monitors are built into some gym equipment. Many women find them fun to use and like the precise, detailed feedback they provide. But you can get the same information without spending any money by taking your radial (wrist) pulse. (Note: don't take your pulse at your neck, by pressing on your carotid artery—that could impede blood flow to your brain.)

To take your radial pulse, all you need is a clock or watch with a second hand.

- Position yourself so you can see your watch or the clock.

- Bend your right arm at the elbow and hold your right hand out.

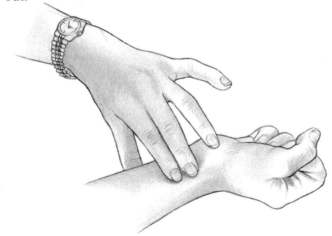

◆ Holding the forefinger and middle finger of your left hand together, touch them to the base of your right thumb.

◆ Very slowly, slide the fingers across your wrist, moving them parallel to the top of your right arm. Your left fingers will cross the bones of your right wrist, then you'll feel a narrow hollow in your right forearm between the bone on top and the tendons below.

◆ Press firmly when you're at the hollow. You should be able to feel your radial pulse. It may help to bend your right wrist back slightly.

◆ Watching the clock, count the number of beats you feel for fifteen seconds. Multiply the number by four to get your heart rate—the number of beats per minute.

During an exercise session, you'll have to slow down a little to check your pulse. This will decrease your heart rate, so practice a few times to get the knack of taking the measurement quickly. Two good times to check your heart rate: when you're five minutes into your aerobic activity, and at the end before you cool down. And you can check it whenever you want to know how hard you're working.

TARGET HEART RATE
FOR AEROBIC EXERCISE

Your **target heart rate** is 60 to 80 percent of your maximum heart rate. During aerobic exercise sessions you'll work out at 60 to 70 percent most of the time, occasionally going up to 75 or 80 percent. Use this formula to estimate your maximum heart rate (or use the chart on the next page):

MAXIMUM HEART RATE = 220 minus your age in years
TARGET HEART RATE = 60 percent to 80 percent of maximum

Example:

Lois is 40. Her maximum heart rate is 180, which is
220 minus 40.

60 percent of 180 (.6 × 180) is 108 beats per minute.

70 percent of 180 (.7 × 180) is 126 beats per minute.

80 percent of 180 (.8 × 180) is 144 beats per minute.

When Lois exercises, she'll maintain a heart rate of 108 to 144 beats
per minute, staying between 108 and 126 most of the time.

TARGET HEART RATE
(BEATS PER MINUTE)

MAINTAIN A HEART RATE BETWEEN 60% AND 80% OF MAXIMUM,
STAYING BETWEEN 60% AND 70% MOST OF THE TIME.

Age	60%	70%	80%	90%
20	120	140	160	180
25	117	137	156	176
30	114	133	152	171
35	111	130	148	167
40	108	126	144	162
45	105	123	140	158
50	102	119	136	153
55	99	116	132	149
60	96	112	128	144
65	93	109	124	140
70	90	105	120	135
75	87	102	116	131
80	84	98	112	126

WHAT ELSE AFFECTS YOUR HEART RATE?

Your heart responds to changes in your activity. As you work harder, it beats faster; when you slow down, your heart slows down too. During outdoor exercise, your heart rate will vary as you go up and down hills or stop for a traffic light. But your heart rate can be affected by other factors as well:

◆ If you're using a pacemaker or taking drugs to keep your heart rate steady.

◆ If you're taking medications that can raise or lower your heart rate, such as cold remedies, appetite suppressants, or calcium channel blockers for blood pressure.

◆ If you've recently consumed caffeine, which can raise your heart rate. Caffeine is found not only in coffee and tea, but also in some sodas and medications.

In these situations, use the exercise intensity scale to assess your effort rather than relying on your pulse. When in doubt, always err on the side of caution and slow your pace. Also, if you have concerns, talk to your doctor.

TEN WEEKS TO AEROBIC FITNESS

As you know by now, I'm a strong believer in the power of slow starts and gradual but steady improvement. Nevertheless, you may be surprised by how little is expected of you at first on the *Strong Women Stay Slim* program: no aerobic exercise for the first two weeks, and just ten minutes the week after that. While this is a slower beginning than some physiologists might advise, there are good reasons to wait.

First, if you've been sedentary, your muscles, tendons, and ligaments may be weak. Two weeks of strength training will make them stronger, so your first aerobic workouts will be easier and safer. Second, there's a lot going on when you start this program: you're learning the strengthening exercises, beginning to keep food records, and changing your diet. I don't want you to ever feel overwhelmed. If you begin gradually and progress steadily, you can painlessly ease yourself into a healthy lifestyle. When you look back ten weeks from now, you'll be astonished and delighted by how far you've come.

How Fit Are You Now? Take the Walking Test

If you can comfortably walk a mile, I encourage you to take the simple walking test below to estimate your aerobic fitness before you begin the program. I developed this test from my experience working with women of different ages and abilities, and by reviewing current medical research on walking and fitness levels. Over the coming weeks and months, you'll be able to repeat the test and track your fitness progress. Here's what to do:

Step 1: Take the Par-Q questionnaire on page 98 to learn if you need to check with your doctor first. If you're very out of shape, or if your mobility is limited by arthritis or another condition, skip the walking test for now. You may be able to take it in a few weeks, after you've gradually increased your strength and cardiovascular fitness.

Step 2: Find a track or a road with a measured mile where walking is safe. If you prefer a track, call your local high school, college, or community center to ask about using the facility; find out how many laps equal a mile.

Step 3: Select a day when the weather is good. Dress as you would for a workout, in comfortable clothes and sturdy shoes. Bring along a stopwatch plus a pencil and paper.

Step 4: Before the test, warm up for five minutes by walking at a moderate pace.

Step 5: Begin the test. Note the time and walk one mile as fast as you comfortably can. If you regularly run or jog, you may do so for all or part of the test.

Step 6: Record your time as you finish the mile.

Step 7: Cool down by walking slowly for five minutes.

Step 8: Check the chart on page 162 to determine your fitness level.

Don't be discouraged if you fall into a low category or can't even complete the test. That's not surprising if you haven't been exercising, especially if you're overweight. If you start working out regularly, you *will* improve—and that will be a great accomplishment. Indeed, just completing the test can be a major achievement for a woman who was extremely sedentary before she started the program.

How to Find the Right Progress Track

Depending on your present fitness, you'll follow one of three different progress tracks. Use the test results, or if you didn't take the test, approximate your level of fitness with the following table:

What's Your Progress Track?

If your FITNESS TEST SCORE IS	Or your FITNESS APPROXIMATION IS	Then your PROGRESS TRACK IS
Excellent or very good	"I can briskly walk, jog, or run a mile."	FAST
Good or fair	"I can walk a mile without resting, but couldn't run or jog."	MEDIUM
Poor or unable to take the test	"I couldn't walk a mile without resting."	SLOW

Aerobic Fitness
Minutes to walk or run a mile

Age	Excellent	Very good	Good	Fair	Poor
20–39	less than 12	12:00–13:59	14:00–15:59	16:00–17:59	18 or more
40–49	less than 13	13:00–14:59	15:00–16:59	17:00–18:59	19 or more
50–59	less than 14	14:00–16:59	17:00–18:59	19:00–20:59	21 or more
60–69	less than 15	15:00–17:59	18:00–19:59	20:00–21:59	22 or more
70 and older	less than 16	16:00–18:59	19:00–20:59	21:00–22:59	23 or more

If you're not sure where you belong on this scale, select the lower category. While going too fast could cause problems, progressing a little less rapidly than you might have is no cause for concern. At the end of ten weeks, you'll be at the same point no matter how quickly you got there.

Remember: if you're already doing aerobic exercise, you don't have to stop. Keep working out at your present level, but pay attention to the intensity level and to the time you spend. At first, you may be far ahead of the weekly progress goals I suggest below, but as time passes, you'll probably find that the goals in the table catch up. From that point on, continue with the *Strong Women Stay Slim* program.

WEEKLY GOALS FOR AEROBIC ACTIVITY

Unless you're already exercising, you don't have to begin aerobic activity until the third week. At that point, you'll do a ten-minute workout at Level 3 intensity, plus warm-up, cool-down, and stretch. Thereafter you'll gradually increase the aerobic sessions to thirty minutes.

If you're already fit, you'll progress more rapidly. Use the chart on the next page to set weekly progress goals, and be sure to keep logs (see pages 215–216) to track your improvement.

Do at least three Level 3 aerobic workouts per week—but no more than six. Your body needs a day of rest. Studies find that people who overdo aerobic exercise by training seven days a week have more injuries than those who take a weekly break.

If you want to do strength training and aerobic activity during the same workout, it's best to do the aerobic exercise first so that your muscles are warmed up. Follow this sequence:

- ♦ Warm-up
- ♦ Aerobic activity
- ♦ Cool-down
- ♦ Strength training
- ♦ Stretches (from Chapter 7 pages 134–137)

I'm frequently asked whether it's okay to break a twenty-minute session into two ten-minute sessions a day. Yes, it is. In fact, the newest research shows that splitting your sessions into ten-minute segments is just as effective for improving cardiovascular fitness. Because you still need to warm up and

Use the chart on page 161 to determine your progress track.

WEEKLY PROGRESS GOALS
MINUTES OF LEVEL 3 AEROBIC ACTIVITY,
THREE TO SIX DAYS PER WEEK

Week	Slow Track	Medium Track	Fast Track
1	0	0	0
2	0	0	0
3	10	10	10
4	10	10	15
5	10	15	20
6	15	15	20
7	15	20	25
8	20	25	30
9	25	30	30
10	30	30	30

cool down for each mini-session, you actually end up exercising more throughout the day.

Which way is best—one long session or several short ones? Your preference should be the deciding factor. Dianne enjoys short walks tucked into her busy day. When she has an appointment near a nice place to walk, she arrives fifteen minutes early so she can take a brisk walk. She builds walking time into everyday errands, such as going to the post office. But Alexandra says, "I like to get into my exercise clothes, work out, shower, and change—and be done with it."

Women also ask if they can move ahead more quickly. A better plan is to increase your Level 2 activity: spend more time walking; cultivate a hobby that gets you moving; take up a sport instead of just watching. You'll burn extra calories and develop a healthier, more vibrant lifestyle. I really enjoy keeping active because it makes me feel so good. So, in addition to my runs, I make a point of walking whenever possible.

HOW YOU'LL FEEL ALONG THE WAY

I urge you to keep exercise logs (see pages 215–216). They will help you stay on track, and later you'll enjoy rereading your early entries and marveling at the improvements. If you've never been physically active before, here's what you can expect over the next ten weeks.

During Weeks 1 to 4

You'll begin aerobic activity by Week 3. Most women I work with see a difference almost immediately, especially if they've been sedentary. First, they feel good about themselves for starting to exercise. They experience a postexercise lift, and often tell me they have more energy throughout the day and sleep better at night.

Because this program starts so gradually, you probably won't experience muscle soreness unless you've been very inactive. When soreness occurs, it usually doesn't develop right away. Instead, you feel it the day after. This is normal; the discomfort should disappear in a day or two. Unless it's severe (which is extremely unlikely), just continue with your workouts. Be sure to warm up, cool down, and stretch, to help your muscles and heart adjust to the exercise.

Some women experience joint pain when they begin an exercise program. This usually doesn't mean they've injured themselves. Usually they're uncovering an existing problem that was masked by inactivity. If this happens to you, progress more slowly and work out at Level 2 intensity instead of Level 3. In a week or two—when you've gotten stronger from strength training and aerobic activity—you should be able to exercise without joint pain.

During Weeks 5 to 10

By now your workouts should be familiar and comfortable. Indeed, I hope they're so enjoyable that you miss them if you have to skip a session.

To maintain Level 3 effort, you've probably stepped up the pace—you're walking a little faster, pedaling your bike a little harder. And you're able to sustain this effort for a longer time. All this is evidence that your body is getting fitter.

If you weren't able to take the walking test at the beginning, perhaps you are ready for it now. If you took the test, retake it when you're halfway through the program. I think you'll be surprised by the progress you've made.

At the End of Week 10

Congratulations! You're exercising thirty minutes a day, at least three days a week—which puts you in the most active quarter of American women. Depending on where you started, your cardiovascular fitness has probably increased by 10 to 20 percent. What's more, you've developed an exercise habit that will keep you fit. Take the walking test again if you can; if you took it before, compare your score with earlier results. I'm sure you'll be very proud to see how far your hard work has taken you.

What's next? You might want to try new activities, or you can stick with what you're doing. As you continue to get fitter, you'll need to adjust your pace to maintain Level 3 effort. Some women are willing to invest the time in longer workouts. That's fine—just be sure to increase gradually, adding no more than five minutes to each session in a week. For example: take at least three weeks to increase your workouts from thirty minutes to forty-five minutes.

BECOMING A MORE ACTIVE PERSON

I've been discussing Level 3 exercise, but I also want to emphasize how important it is—for weight reduction, for your health, and for your emotional well-being—to be more active throughout the day. Here are a few suggestions:

- **Use yourself for transportation.** Instead of taking the shuttle bus at work, I walk the eight blocks from the parking garage to my office. When I'm running errands on the weekend, I walk the mile-and-a-half to town rather than using the car. This doesn't take a lot of time—in fact, sometimes I actually save time by walking.

- **Adopt active hobbies.** Try new sports; go dancing; take up gardening.

- **Socialize on the move.** Instead of meeting a friend for lunch, take a walk together. Play active games with your family.

- **Cultivate inefficiency.** Labor-saving devices keep you from burning calories! Rake the leaves instead of using an electric blower; if you live in a house with stairs, make a point of going up and down as often as possible.

ACTIVITIES

The easiest way to develop an exercise habit is to select an activity that's readily available and that you enjoy (or at least consider tolerable). Some people, including me, love to get outdoors to exercise. They want to breathe fresh air; they want to go places and see the countryside. Others prefer indoor workouts, for different but equally valid reasons. They don't have to worry about the weather, traffic, or unsafe neighborhoods, and they can use exercise machines, which help calibrate effort. Either way is fine. I suggest you focus on one or two activities during the first ten weeks.

To help you decide, I'll discuss popular options that are particularly well suited to beginners. The list is by no means complete. If you belong to a gym, you may have access to many exercise machines, not just the few I've described. Anything that allows you to work at the right intensity, while feeling comfortable and safe, is good to use. A fitness instructor at the gym can help you get started.

You may be surprised that my list doesn't include tennis, squash, volleyball, or other competitive sports. These are terrific, enjoyable activities—if you're already doing them, just continue. Otherwise I don't recommend them for your "daily bread" workouts at this point. First, most of these activities aren't available every day, which is so important when you're trying to establish an exercise habit. In addition, they require bursts of activity plus sudden side movements, which are hard on your body unless you're already fit. So get in shape first, and then get involved in sports.

WALKING

Walking is often called the ideal aerobic exercise—and for good reason. Most of your muscles, as well as your cardiovascular system, get a workout when you walk. Walking tones your leg muscles. It's also great for weight control: it can use up a lot of calories, and it helps burn fat in the abdominal area.

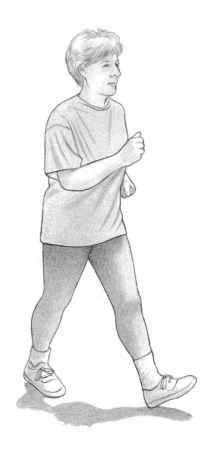

If you walk outdoors, there's no need to purchase special equipment other than good shoes. Just be conscious of the outside temperature, and make sure your clothing is appropriate. An added convenience: you can tuck walking into your everyday routine, so you don't need to set aside much extra time for exercise.

Maintain good posture and swing your arms comfortably. As you become fitter, you'll need to increase intensity to maintain Level 3 effort. One way to do this is to walk faster. But once you reach three and a half to four miles per hour—a very brisk walk— you'd have to jog or run, which is harder on your joints. If you want to break into a jog or run, I suggest you wait until you've been exercising for at least ten weeks; this reduces the risk of orthopedic problems. In the meantime, you can reach Level 3 effort by walking uphill.

Some women increase intensity by carrying dumbbells or wearing wrist weights when they walk. If you've done this and feel you benefit, you can continue. But I don't recommend it. Adding weight can throw off your gait and balance, which could lead to joint problems. I think it's better to increase effort by going uphill or moving faster.

For those who'd rather walk indoors, treadmills are very popular. Use an electric treadmill rather than the kind powered by your movement. (Non-electric treadmills are more difficult to start and walk on, so it's harder to get a good workout. Also, they can be unsteady.) Look for a treadmill that's easy

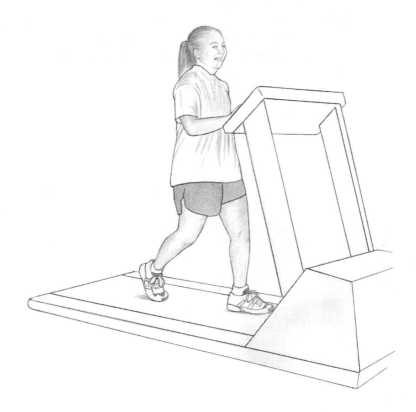

to adjust. The belt should be wide enough so you feel steady when you walk. Make sure the walking surface is long enough for your stride, even if you move forward or back a little. Also important for safety are handrails on the side or front.

The first few times you use a treadmill, you may feel unsteady even if you don't normally have problems with balance. I suggest you gently hold on to the handrail until you're more comfortable. But as soon as you're able, try to walk without holding on because you'll have a better workout and burn more calories. Swing your arms and stride as you would if you were walking on the ground, with your heel striking the ground first. If you work out at a gym, ask a fitness instructor to check your form. To help maintain balance, find a focal point—something to look at that's straight ahead and about ten to twenty feet away. If you need to turn your head, don't just spin around; hold the handrail and turn slowly.

As you lose weight and become fitter, you may find that you no longer reach Level 3 intensity. Adjustments are simple on the treadmill, since you can set the speed and incline. Try both kinds of increases to see which you prefer. However, during the first ten weeks, don't use an incline above 5 percent.

Some treadmills (and other exercise machines) have built-in programs that simulate walks over hilly terrain. While this feature is fun to use and adds variety to your workout, it may force you to work at an intensity that's too high or too low. Therefore, I suggest you stick with a fixed intensity for the first few weeks. After you're fitter you can experiment with different programs.

CYCLING

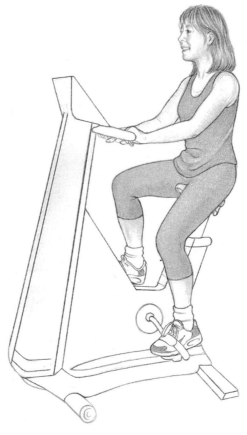

Biking and stationary cycling are also excellent exercises. Pedaling burns a lot of calories, and it works the muscles in your lower body. Cycling is great for your abs and it firms your bottom. Another important advantage is that it's easy on your joints. Also, many women find aerobic activity more enjoyable when they can do it sitting down. Cycling is a great way to have fun and go places—and it's something to do with your family.

Stationary cycles come in different forms: upright, like an ordinary bicycle, or semi-recumbent, with a back to lean on for support. Most cycles train only the lower body, but some include an arm element that works the upper body. You might find those a bit difficult to use at first, since they require coordination. If so, start on a regular stationary cycle and focus on giving your legs a good workout.

When you buy a bicycle or stationary cycle, ask the sales person (or fitness instructor if you're at a gym) to help you get a good fit. The handlebars should be a comfortable distance in front, so your arms are neither cramped

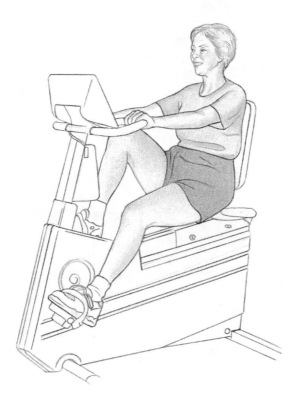

nor stretched out. Proper seat adjustment is also important. Adjust the height so that when your foot is flat on the pedal and the pedal is pushed all the way down, your knee is just slightly bent. You should feel comfortably balanced on the seat—experiment with the pitch, tilting it slightly forward or back, until you find a good position.

If you're using a stationary cycle, set the resistance so you can pedal at a rate of 55 to 65 revolutions per minute. As with the treadmill, I don't recommend using the built-in programs that simulate hills until you've been exercising for several weeks. Two safety precautions: select clothing that won't get caught in the gears or wheels, and if you ride outdoors, always wear a helmet.

CROSS-COUNTRY SKIING

Cross-country skiing is an ideal aerobic exercise. It trains major muscles in the upper and lower body, and doesn't put a lot of strain on the joints. The entire trunk of your body—back, abs, and shoulders—will be firmer. Once you learn the move—and it can be tricky at first—you'll find cross-country skiing as easy as walking. Unfortunately, most of us don't live in lo-

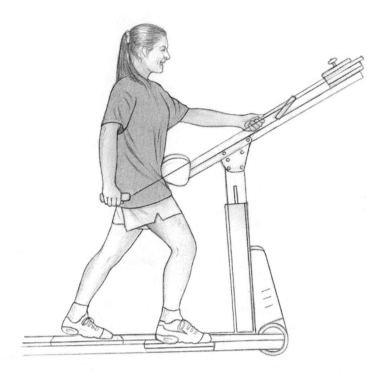

cations that allow this to be our "daily bread" activity. But because cross-country skiing is such a superb fitness activity, exercise machines have been developed to simulate the movements.

Ski machines are getting better and better. If you tried one a long time ago and didn't like it, give them another chance. Look for a machine that lets you adjust leg and arm resistance independently; some also let you increase the slope. With a little experimenting, you'll find the right settings.

Expect to spend a few sessions learning how to work the skis. It might help to hold on to the handles and do just the leg move at first. When you've mastered that, add the arm motion.

ROWING

Like cross-country skiing, rowing works your upper and lower body (including your abs), but it doesn't strain your joints. This is another superb exercise that's more practical for most of us in its simulated form.

When you select a machine, check that the seat and "oars" (the bar you pull back) move very smoothly. I much prefer flywheel rowers to the hydraulic piston variety; I find the movement much smoother and more like real rowing. For safety, make sure the flywheel is encased.

The resistance and the stroke rate needn't be high to give you a great workout. Aim for 26 to 30 strokes per minute. Each stroke has two parts. First, you pull the oars toward your body and stretch out your legs to push the seat away from the flywheel, making sure not to lock your knees. Second, stretch your arms forward, and bend your knees to bring the seat back toward the flywheel; your arms need to go past your knees before they bend. Try to make the movement smooth and fluid.

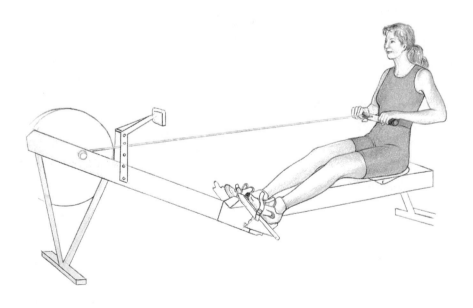

STAIR CLIMBING

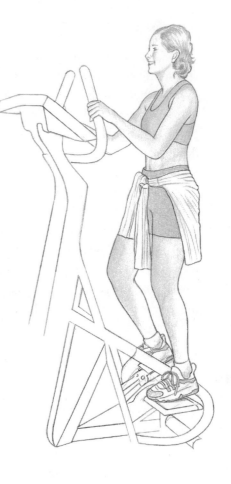

Stair climbing is a terrific aerobic activity that some people, including me, find easy to fit into their lives. My office is on the fourteenth floor of a high-rise building. At least a couple of times a week, I make a point of using the stairs instead of the elevator. This isn't my "daily bread" activity, because it takes just five minutes. But it's a terrific stress-reducer.

Some athletes do stair-climbing workouts in outdoor stadiums, but for most people a stair-climbing machine is more practical. This very popular device provides great aerobic exercise, and it conditions the lower legs, abdomen, back, thighs, and calves. But stair climbers are not for everyone. If you have bad knees and can't comfortably use a regular stair climber, try a semi-recumbent model, which supports your body weight as you work out. Also, since stair climbers can elevate your heart rate very quickly, especially if you're heavy, progress gradually if you're out of shape.

Select a model that has a very smooth stepping action. The foot plates should be wide and secure enough to hold your foot steady without wobbling, and the handlebars should be easy to hold. Take natural steps; the ankle of your "up" foot should be between the calf and knee of your "down" foot; this generally means about eight to ten inches.

Good posture is important. Stand tall and hold the rails lightly, just for balance. A common mistake is to grip the handrails and lean on them for support. But if you do that, your legs aren't getting a full workout. If you can't keep up the pace in good form, that's a sign that you need to go slower or ease the resistance a bit.

CLASSES AND VIDEOS

Aerobics classes are a delightful way to work out. The moves can involve everything from dancing to boxing; some classes use equipment, including steps and weights. You may find a "spinning" class in which a trainer leads the group on a simulated bike ride through the country.

Talk with the instructor before you select a class. Make sure the required fitness level is appropriate for you—not too demanding, but sufficiently challenging so you'll have a Level 3 workout. For instance, step aerobics can be overly strenuous if you're out of shape or have knee problems. Chose a low-impact workout, where one foot is on the floor at all times, since this greatly lowers the risk of joint injuries. The class should include periods for warm-up, cool-down, and stretching.

What about "toning" aerobics classes that use light weights? They're fine if the aerobic intensity level is right for you. Just realize that you're only working your cardiovascular system, because light weights will *not* increase your strength.

Exercise videos let you bring some of the fun of an aerobics class into your home. Read the box carefully to get the information an instructor would have provided. If possible, rent a video before you buy, to make sure it's appropriate and enjoyable.

SWIMMING AND AQUA AEROBICS

Swimming is an excellent exercise. You get an aerobic workout and also train major muscles in your upper and lower body. It's particularly appropriate for women with arthritis or orthopedic problems, since your weight is supported by water. Learn different strokes—freestyle, breast stroke, and back stroke—to vary your routine and strengthen different muscles. Just be aware that it's a little harder to gauge intensity when you're in the water since you're not sweating, so learn to take your pulse.

Another popular water activity is aqua aerobics. Led by a well-trained instructor, you can get an excellent, enjoyable workout that's easy on your joints because the water helps support your weight. Sometimes when I suggest aqua aerobics, a woman will confess that she feels self-conscious about putting on a bathing suit. But most classes have a wider range of body types than you'd expect, and participants have a great time once they're in the water.

9

A LIFELONG PLAN

FOR EATING WELL

I used to count calories rather than look at the kind of food I was eating. My diet didn't add up to good nutrition. I wasn't losing weight, even though I was skipping meals. I've cut down on portions. I'm aware when I've had enough protein and when I need to eat something with calcium. If I'm hungry, I have a fruit or a vegetable. Over six months I've lost nineteen pounds. It hasn't been that difficult because I have had plenty to eat.
　　—Nancy

◆　◆　◆

The *Strong Women Stay Slim* food plan is not a temporary diet that you'll force yourself to endure for a few months, then abandon with enormous relief after you lose weight. This plan will become a valuable part of your life. It's based on the USDA Food Pyramid, which represents the best up-to-the-minute information from the nation's leading experts on nutrition and health. I've used it with dozens of women—not only the volunteers in my research projects, but also friends and relatives who want to lose weight. I can assure you that it really works. The plan is health-promoting, flexible, and practical. You can follow it if you're traveling and eating in restaurants, if you're a vegetarian, if you have food allergies, or if you observe religious dietary restrictions.

Losing weight is just one of the benefits. Women who haven't been eating well are astonished by how good they feel when they're well nourished. They're more energetic and alert throughout the day. Gone are the sluggishness and the cranky low periods. Best of all, they're so pleased and proud of what they're doing for themselves.

THE POWER OF POSITIVE EATING

This food plan emphasizes what you *should* eat, not what you *shouldn't* eat. Because good nutrition is so important, it's as much a mistake to skip a meal or omit a fruit as it is to have extra dessert.

TAKE TIME TO ENJOY

Eating good food is one of the great pleasures of life, so take the time to sit down and savor your meals. I realize this can be a challenge. If you're running errands at lunchtime, it's tempting to grab a sandwich and eat in the car. And many a weary mother has made a meal of her children's leftovers, consumed as she carries their plates from the table to the kitchen sink. But the time invested in preparing a wholesome dinner, setting the table, relaxing, and eating slowly really pays off. You'll find your meals much more satisfying, and that will help you stick with the food plan.

EAT WHATEVER YOU WANT— IN REASONABLE QUANTITY

There are no forbidden foods on this plan. You can have breads, pasta, eggs, red meat—and even butter, ice cream, and chocolate. After all, people who are naturally thin eat these foods. Of course, you'll have to limit the amount if you want to lose weight. But if you eat slowly, and concentrate on enjoying each mouthful, a modest serving can be very satisfying.

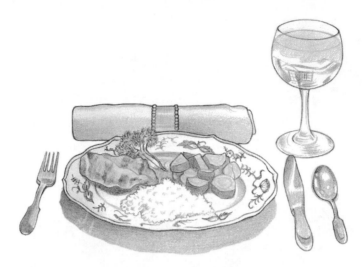

COUNT PORTIONS, NOT CALORIES

On this plan, you'll track portions and types of food—dairy, grain, fruit, and so on—not calories. I prefer this system for two reasons. First, it's easy to use. You won't have to remember lots of details. Second, it promotes variety, a key to a healthy, well-balanced diet.

Note that I'm *not* saying that calories don't count—they definitely do! I'll refer to calories occasionally in this chapter; you may need to check calories if you want to add a food I haven't listed. But most of the time, you don't have to think about calories. If you follow the plan, you'll automatically be eating the correct amount.

FIVE SIMPLE RULES THAT MINIMIZE HUNGER AND MAXIMIZE ENERGY

When you're well nourished—when your body has enough food and all the nutrients it needs—it's easier to lose weight. Your appetite is satisfied, so you aren't derailed by hunger and cravings. You have energy throughout the day. Finally, you can get off the blood-sugar roller coaster that leaves you desperate and irritable at some times, and groggy and bloated at others.

Here are five rules that optimize the nutritional payoff when you're following this food plan:

#1: EAT AT LEAST THREE MEALS A DAY

Your body and mind perform best with a steady supply of food. I often see a vicious circle that starts when a woman doesn't take time for breakfast. On the way to work she gulps a cup of coffee—she's kick-starting her engine, but she hasn't given it any fuel. Things get worse because she's too busy for lunch. By late afternoon, she's been fasting for twenty hours. Not surprisingly, she's ravenous and has trouble thinking clearly. She figures that since she hasn't eaten all day, she doesn't have to limit herself now. So on the way home she picks up a drive-through dinner that's high on fat but low on other nutrients. The next morning, still feeling the effects of the night before, she skips breakfast—and the whole situation repeats itself.

I strongly recommend that you eat three meals a day. You can also have one or more snacks, as you prefer. Some women get hungry between meals; for them, two or three snacks work well. Other women find that snacks actually make them hungrier, so they eat just at mealtime. I never get hungry between meals when I'm at work, but I like to have a snack when I get home, to take the edge off my hunger as I prepare dinner.

◆ ◆ ◆

I was a reckless, chaotic eater. I never planned. Some days I didn't eat anything until three-thirty in the afternoon. I was hungry without realizing it. It was important for me to stabilize my eating and develop a regular meal plan.
—Dianne

◆ ◆ ◆

Sometimes women who are planning a special event ask me if they can "bank" calories—eat less than their daily plan permits for several days, so they can splurge later on. This is something I don't advise. Your body is working all the time, and it needs food to function optimally. You're much less likely to overeat at a special event if you've been well nourished throughout the week. If you arrive semistarved, you'll find it more difficult to stay in control.

#2: INCLUDE AT LEAST THREE FOOD GROUPS AT EVERY MEAL

Your body needs carbohydrates and protein, and there's some evidence that your energy improves if you consume them together. Though this hasn't been extensively researched, my experience and that of other nutritionists suggests that people perform better if they eat a variety of foods throughout the day. Variety also makes for more interesting and satisfying meals. For instance, your sliced chicken sandwich will seem more like a complete lunch if you also have a piece of fruit. You may not be able to include three food groups at every meal, but I encourage you to try, especially at your main meal of the day.

#3: GO FOR A RAINBOW OF FRUITS AND VEGETABLES

Fruits and vegetables are low in calories and high in nutrients, which makes them ideal foods for weight loss. Nature has color-coded them. For example, dark green vegetables are rich in calcium and folate; orange vegetables contain carotene, which your body converts to vitamin A. Therefore, a simple way to assure you're getting a healthy variety of nutrients is to enjoy an attractive mix of colors.

◆ ◆ ◆

I used to serve one vegetable with dinner; now I usually serve three. One of my favorite combinations in the winter is steamed broccoli, baked buttercup squash, and red cabbage. The colors are beautiful: green, bright orange, and deep purple. If there were just one vegetable, I wouldn't eat three portions. But if there's a variety, I do. This makes the meal much more filling. It's not a lot of work, because I choose vegetables that are simple to prepare, or I buy them ready-to-cook from the salad bar.
—Sarah

◆ ◆ ◆

#4: SELECT WHOLE GRAINS

Try to consume at least half of the day's grains in unprocessed form—whole wheat bread instead of white bread, brown rice instead of white. After grains are processed, manufacturers enrich them in an effort to restore lost nutrients. However, the enriched versions contain very little fiber, trace minerals, and other components of whole grains. Because of their fiber content, whole grains are digested more slowly than processed versions, so they keep your appetite satisfied longer.

#5: DRINK PLENTY OF FLUIDS

Your body needs to be well hydrated to function at its best. Most people are chronically underhydrated because they don't drink enough. This is often an unsuspected factor in lethargy, fatigue, dry skin, and constipation. You may be surprised at how much better you look and feel when you start drinking more. Also, fluid is one of the great weight-loss aids. Sipping a beverage along with a meal or snack will help you feel satisfied sooner. Liquids also improve the performance of your digestive and metabolic systems.

Try to drink at least eight cups of fluids a day, especially water. Alco-

A SIMPLE PRECAUTION

If you're following this plan, you're probably getting all the nutrients you need. Still, just as a precaution, take a multivitamin and mineral supplement. Standard supplements contain 100 percent of the RDA (Recommended Dietary Allowance) for the essential vitamins, and 25 to 100 percent of the RDA for a variety of minerals. Check the label to make sure the supplement supplies vitamins D and E, as well as folate and calcium—these are the nutrients many people miss in their diets, even if they eat well. If your multivitamin doesn't include calcium, consider a daily calcium supplement that contains 300 milligrams (if you're premenopausal) to 500 milligrams (if you're postmenopausal); this will complement the calcium in your diet. Note: another option is to get extra nutrients from fortified foods, such as vitamin-fortified breakfast cereals or orange juice with added calcium.

holic and caffeinated beverages don't count because they stimulate the kidneys to increase urine volume, a dehydrating effect.

YOU CAN EAT MORE THAN YOU THOUGHT YOU COULD— AND STILL LOSE WEIGHT

The healthiest way to lose weight—and the best way to establish habits that will keep it off—is to eat a well-balanced diet that trims calories just enough to let you lose one or two pounds a week. Many diet books put all women on 1000 to 1200 calories per day, no matter how active they are and no matter how much they weigh. But if you're doing strength training and aerobic exercise, you may be able to lose weight on 1600 to 2000 calories a day.

WHICH LEVEL IS RIGHT FOR YOU?

You've already learned how to adjust your exercise sessions so you gradually progress toward fitness goals. In the same way, you'll calibrate your food consumption so you lose between one and two pounds per week. If you lose too quickly, you'll eat a little more; if you lose too slowly, you'll have a little less. After you reach your weight goal, similar adjustments will maintain your weight—and you'll know exactly how to make them.

For simplicity, I've included detailed information for three daily calorie levels: 1200, 1600, and 2000. Over time, you'll probably follow more than one of these plans.

HOW TO FIND YOUR STARTING POINT

The best way to determine a good starting point—what you'd do if you were working individually with a nutritionist—is to keep a food diary for a week to find out how many calories you're consuming now. You'd then aim for a food plan that provides about 500 calories per day less than what you usually eat. This would let you lose one to two pounds a week if you're also exercising.

While you could do similar calculations on your own, most women can use the simple table on page 183 to arrive at an appropriate starting point.

IF YOUR GOAL IS	YOUR PRELIMINARY STARTING LEVEL IS
To lose up to 100 pounds	1600 calories
To lose 100 pounds or more	2000 calories
To maintain your current weight, but improve your eating habits	2000 calories

Two exceptions:

- If you are already very physically active, start at 2000 calories even if you plan to lose less than 100 pounds.

- If you've been following a very stringent diet that provides much less food than the *Strong Women Stay Slim* plan recommends, and your weight is currently stable, decrease to the next lower calorie level—from 2000 to 1600, or from 1600 to 1200.

Don't worry if you're uncertain which level is best—this is just the beginning. Once you're following the plan and see how it works, you can easily adjust as needed.

THREE DAILY PLANS

The chart lists types of food and suggests the number of daily portions for three different calorie levels: 1200, 1600, and 2000. Following the chart are lists of specific foods, so you'll know how much a portion is.

The calorie counts are merely averages. One woman who meticulously follows the 1600-calorie plan may wind up eating closer to 1500 calories, because she happens to select lower-calorie items from the food list; another, just as careful, might consume nearly 1700 calories because her choices are consistently at the top of the range.

THE DAILY FOOD PLANS

FOOD GROUP	NUMBER OF PORTIONS EACH DAY		
	1200 CALORIES	1600 CALORIES	2000 CALORIES
Dairy: milk, yogurt, cheese, soy equivalents	2	3	3
Protein: meat, poultry, fish, beans, tofu, eggs, nuts	4	5	6
Grain: bread, cereal, rice, pasta	5	6	8
Vegetable	3	4	5
Fruit	2	3	4
Extras: fats, oils, sweets	4	6	8

WHAT IS A PORTION?

'll use the word **portion** to mean a prescribed amount of a particular food. As you'll see, it's often not the amount you'd think of as a normal **serving**, which is the amount you'd put on your plate. For example, one portion of pasta is just half a cup. If you have pasta for dinner, your serving might be two or three Grain portions. A four-ounce serving of boneless chicken counts as four Protein portions.

Some items count as more than one food group. For example, a roast beef sandwich made from two slices of bread and two ounces of roast beef would be two Grains for the bread and two Proteins for the meat.

Certain foods are higher in sugar or fat, so they contain more calories per portion than typical for their group. To compensate, these items draw upon your allotment of Extras. For example, if you have a half cup of low-fat frozen yogurt, that counts as a Dairy portion plus one Extra; if you have four ounces of spareribs, that's four Proteins plus two Extras. I've tried to list most common foods, but some of your favorites may be missing. If you can obtain calorie information (for instance, by reading a food label), you can figure out portion equivalents.

PORTIONS OR CALORIES?

One reason I prefer to count portions rather than calories is that outside the laboratory, it's really impossible to determine calories precisely. I'm always amused when I see overly precise calorie counts—like "453 calories per serving" on a recipe for vegetable lasagna. Was the grated cheese densely or loosely packed? Were all the servings cut exactly the same size or were some half-an-inch wider than others? In reality, that "453-calorie" lasagna serving could contain anywhere from around 400 to 500 or more calories.

When you start using the food plan, you'll need to check the lists frequently, and the calculations may seem complex. But I promise you that in a week or two everything will be much easier. The Portion Primer that starts on page 195 will be very helpful.

Dairy (or Equivalents)

Dairy foods are very rich in high-quality protein, calcium (which is especially important for women), vitamin D (in the case of milk), riboflavin, and other vitamins and minerals. But most dairy products are also naturally high in saturated fat. Fortunately, there are excellent low- or non-fat versions. If you use them, you won't miss out on any nutrients. In fact, a portion of skim milk actually has a little more calcium than whole milk. If you prefer soy or rice milk, check the label to make sure it's fortified with calcium.

Milk, whole	1 cup (plus 2 Extras)
Milk, 1 to 2 percent fat	1 cup (plus 1 Extra)
Milk, non-fat	1 cup
Soy or rice milk, with fat	1 cup (plus 1 Extra)
Soy or rice milk, non-fat	1 cup
Yogurt, whole milk (plain or flavored)	1 cup (plus 2 Extras)
Yogurt, low-fat	1 cup (plus 1 Extra)
Yogurt, non-fat	1 cup
Cottage cheese, whole milk	1/2 cup (plus 2 Extras)
Cottage cheese, low-fat	1/2 cup (plus 1 Extra)
Cottage cheese, non-fat	1/2 cup
Ricotta cheese, whole milk	2 ounces (plus 2 Extras)
Ricotta cheese, part skim	2 ounces (plus 1 Extra)
Ricotta cheese, non-fat	2 ounces
Hard cheese (cheddar, Swiss)	1 ounce (plus 1 Extra)
Hard cheese, low- or non-fat	1 ounce
American cheese, regular	1 slice (plus 1 Extra)
American cheese, low- or non-fat	1 slice
Ice cream, regular	1/2 cup (plus 2 Extras)
Ice cream, low- or non-fat	1/2 cup (plus 1 Extra)
Frozen yogurt, low- or non-fat	1/2 cup (plus 1 Extra)
Pudding, low- or non-fat	1/2 cup (plus 1 Extra)

A Dairy portion contains 90 to 120 calories. If you select a dairy food that's high in fat, such as ice cream or whole milk, you'll count the food as a Dairy portion plus two Extra portions; low-fat dairy foods count as a Dairy plus one Extra.

PROTEIN

Meat, poultry, fish, beans, eggs, tofu, and nuts are important sources of protein, iron (especially red meat), zinc, and several B vitamins. Like dairy foods, meats naturally contain fat. Therefore, it's best to choose the leanest cuts and to prepare them with as little added fat as possible. Notice that portions of most fish and tofu are twice as large as a portion of even lean meat or

Poultry, light meat without skin	1 ounce
Poultry, light meat with skin	1 ounce (plus ½ Extra)
Poultry, dark meat without skin	1 ounce (plus ½ Extra)
Poultry, dark meat with skin	1 ounce (plus 1 Extra)
Beef, lean (round, loin, flank)	1 ounce
Beef (chuck, hamburger)	1 ounce (plus ½ Extra)
Hot dog	1 ounce (plus ½ Extra)
Pork, lean (tenderloin, round)	1 ounce
Pork (chops, spareribs)	1 ounce (plus ½ Extra)
Lamb, lean (leg)	1 ounce
Lamb (chops)	1 ounce (plus ½ Extra)
Deli meat or poultry, low-fat	1 ounce
Deli meat, regular	1 ounce (plus ½ Extra)
Fish, light-colored (flounder, cod)	2 ounces
Fish, dark-colored (salmon, bluefish)	1 ounce
Seafood (shrimp, scallops, clams)	2 ounces
Cooked beans (kidney, lima, lentils, chickpeas, pinto)	½ cup
Hummus (chickpea spread)	2 tablespoons
Egg	1 (plus 1 Extra)
Egg whites	3
Egg substitute	½ cup
Tofu	2 ounces
Nuts	1 ounce or 3 tablespoons (plus 1 Extra)
Peanut butter	1 tablespoon (plus 2 Extras)

poultry. I encourage you to try tofu. As I mentioned in Chapter 4, soy products offer very important health benefits for women.

Each Protein portion contains 45 to 80 calories. If you select higher-fat foods, you'll have to compensate with Extras.

GRAINS

Grains, especially whole grains, are indeed the staff of life—the foundation of your diet. These foods are rich in B vitamins, minerals, complex carbohydrates, and fiber. Along with fruits and vegetables, they make your meals more enjoyable and filling.

Try to select unprocessed whole grains for at least half of your Grain allotment—brown rice, oats, barley, cracked wheat. If you're buying bread, look for "whole wheat flour" on the label. Don't assume that peasant-style loaves or "wheat flour" breads are made from whole grains. Often they're pre-

Bread	1 slice (1 ounce)
Pita	1 ounce (1 very small round or ½ of a regular round)
Bagel	½ small bagel (1 ounce)
English muffin	½
Hot dog or hamburger bun	½
Dinner roll	1 small (1 ounce)
Cooked rice	½ cup
Cooked pasta	½ cup
Tortilla	6-inch round
Crackers (saltine type)	5
Croutons	⅓ cup
Pretzels	1 ounce
Chips, nonfat	1 ounce
Popcorn, air-popped	3 cups
Rice cakes	2
Cooked cereal	½ cup
Cold cereal, unsweetened	1 cup
Cold cereal, lightly sweetened	1 cup (plus 1 Extra)
Cold cereal, sweetened	1 cup (plus 2 Extras)
Granola	¼ cup

pared with white flour to which molasses or a small amount of whole wheat flour has been added for color.

Each Grain portion has 60 to 100 calories. Note that some ready-to-eat cereals contain added fat and sugar. Though these can be reasonable choices, especially as substitutes for cookies or cake, they count as Extras as well as Grains.

VEGETABLES

Vegetables provide many vitamins, minerals, health-promoting phytochemicals, and fiber. Most are naturally low in fat and calories. Consume a variety of vegetables to get nature's own multivitamin. Each vegetable portion contains approximately 10 to 40 calories, the lowest of all the food groups.

Cooked green vegetables, carrots, squash, eggplant, mushrooms, red cabbage, cauliflower	½ cup
Lettuce, raw cabbage, or raw spinach	2 cups
Sprouts	1 cup
Raw vegetables, chopped or sliced	½ cup
Artichoke	½ of medium artichoke
Asparagus	6 spears
Avocado	¼ cup (plus 2 Extras)
Brussels sprouts	4 cooked
Carrot	1 medium; 6 baby carrots
Celery stalks	4
Corn	½ ear; ¼ cup kernels
Peas	¼ cup
Tomato	1 whole; ½ cup chopped
Onion	1 whole; ½ cup chopped
Potato, baked with skin	½ small potato
Potato, mashed (include Extras if mashed with butter or sour cream)	¼ cup
Sweet potato with skin	½ small potato
Vegetable juice	6 ounces
Vegetable soup	1 cup
Tomato sauce	½ cup
Salsa (made without oil)	3 tablespoons

FRUITS

Luscious fruits, along with vegetables, contribute numerous vitamins, minerals, and phytochemicals to your diet. Citrus fruits are especially good sources of vitamin C; they also contain some calcium. In addition, the fiber in fruit fills you up and keeps your digestive system moving. As you cut back on empty-calorie desserts and snacks, you'll find the sweetness of fruit more satisfying. A portion of fruit contains 80 to 100 calories.

Fruit (apple, orange, kiwi, peach, nectarine)	1 medium
Fresh fruit, diced	1/2 cup
Fruit, canned in unsweetened juice	1/2 cup
Fruit, canned in sweetened juice	1/2 cup (plus 1 Extra)
Fruit juice (100% juice)	6 ounces
Banana	1 small
Grapefruit	1/2
Plums	2
Apricots	4
Figs	2
Mango	1/2
Melon, diced	1 cup
Berries, cherries, grapes	1 cup if whole, 1/2 cup if sliced
Coconut, fresh	2" by 2" by 1/2" (plus 2 Extras)
Coconut, dry	1 ounce (plus 2 Extras)
Dried fruit	1/4 cup
Dried apple rings	4
Raisins	2 tablespoons

EXTRAS

The list of foods in this category may surprise you since it includes butter, oil, whipped cream, candy, sugar, and other items that many diet plans exclude. Most nutritionists would not consider them a food group, but I'm adding them for several reasons.

First, as you've already seen, this category helps you keep track when you select higher-calorie options from the other groups. For instance, a glass of whole milk counts as one Dairy portion plus two Extras. Added fat is also in this category. In limited quantity, fat is actually useful when you're trying to lose weight. It carries flavor, and because it's broken down more slowly than protein or carbohydrate, fat helps you feel full longer after a meal. Similarly, controlled amounts of sugar can make your food plan more flexible and appealing. And, of course, many people enjoy alcoholic beverages. (Some research suggests that the flavonoids in red wine are health-promoting.)

An Extra portion contains 30 to 70 calories. Remember, some of your daily Extras may come from your selections in the other food groups.

Vegetable and olive oil	1 teaspoon
Butter, margarine, regular mayonnaise (use sparingly because of saturated fats and trans fatty acids)	1 teaspoon
Diet margarine	2 teaspoons
Cream cheese, regular	1 tablespoon
Cream cheese, low- or non-fat	2 tablespoons
Cream, whipped	1 tablespoon
Sour cream, regular	1 tablespoon
Sour cream, low- or non-fat	2 tablespoons
Salad dressing, regular	2 teaspoons
Salad dressing, low-fat	4 teaspoons
Sugar, brown sugar, honey, sweet syrup, jam, jelly, chocolate syrup	2 teaspoons
Midget candy bar	1
Solid chocolate	1/2 ounce
Hard candy, cough drop	3
Cookie, 1 to 2 inches in diameter	1
Animal crackers	7
Graham crackers	3
Biscotti	1/2
Chips, fried (potato, tortilla, etc.)	1/3 ounce (about 5 chips)
Chips, baked (potato, tortilla, etc.)	1/2 ounce (about 8 chips)
Soda	6 ounces
Beer, regular	6 ounces
Beer, light	12 ounces
Wine	6 ounces
Liquor (gin, vodka, scotch, etc.)	1 ounce
Sweet liqueurs	1/2 ounce

WHAT ABOUT SOUPS, CASSEROLES, AND OTHER MULTI-INGREDIENT FOODS?

After a few weeks on this food plan, you'll be able to glance at a plate and know that it contains about three ounces of chicken (three Proteins), one cup of rice (two Grains), and a half-cup of sliced carrots (one Vegetable). But suppose you're at a dinner party, and the hostess serves a seafood pasta casserole in a cheese sauce. How should you count your serving?

Short of requesting a recipe plus measuring utensils, all you can do is guess. Make a quick mental list of ingredients, then estimate portion sizes. For instance, you might figure that your serving of seafood casserole includes about a cup of pasta (two Grains), approximately four ounces of seafood (two Proteins), some chopped vegetables (one Vegetable), plus about half a cup of creamy sauce (call it a half Dairy plus two Extras).

What if you're wrong? Provided you aren't consistently underestimating your consumption, day after day, it really doesn't matter if you're slightly too high or too low at one meal. Do your best, then relax and enjoy the party.

Here are a few examples of combination foods:

Cheese pizza: ⅛ of 12-inch pie	1 Grain, 1½ Dairy, 2 Extras
Pepperoni pizza: ⅛ of 12-inch pie	1 Grain, 1½ Dairy, 1 Protein, 3 Extras
Cheeseburger: 4-ounce burger	2 Grains, 1 Dairy, 4 Proteins, 3 Extras
Macaroni and cheese: 1 cup	2 Grains, 1½ Dairy, 3 Extras
Fruit pie: ⅛ of 9-inch pie	1 Fruit, 1 Grain, 3 Extras
Chocolate layer cake: ¹/₁₂ of 9-inch 2-layer cake with frosting	1 Grain, 4 Extras

THE NEXT-TO-NOTHING LIST

To simplify the plan and give you added flexibility, I've compiled a list of foods that are so low in calories, or used in such small quantities, that you don't have to count them. This means that when you're enjoying a turkey sandwich topped with lettuce and tomato, seasoned with mustard, accompanied by a few dill pickle slices, and garnished with parsley—that's just two Grains for the roll and three Proteins for the turkey.

The Next-to-Nothing (NTN) list is also your insurance against hunger. Use it for snacks and to expand meals. Note: I called this list "*Next-to-Nothing*" for a reason. Most items on the list contain a few calories. So I want to caution you that you could undermine your efforts if you eat very large quantities—that's why I've placed daily limits on certain foods.

You may be puzzled to see some items on the NTN list that are also on the Vegetable list. These can be counted either way. For instance, if you're hungry and want more vegetables than your food plan calls for, have a plate of sliced cucumber, green pepper, and jicama—and record the whole snack as NTN. But if you're behind on vegetables, and need another portion to reach your daily quota, you could count the same snack as a Vegetable.

BEVERAGES

> Water
> Seltzer, club soda
> Diet soda and diet drink mixes
> Coffee
> Tea
> Bouillon, broth (1 cup; may be high in salt)

SAUCES, SEASONINGS, GARNISHES, AND CONDIMENTS

> Garlic
> Mustard
> Fresh ginger
> Horseradish
> Soy sauce, teriyaki sauce
> Hot sauce
> Worcestershire sauce
> Vinegar
> Lemon juice, lime juice
> Nonstick spray
> Herbs and spices (basil, cinnamon, curry, dill, oregano, etc.)
> Flavor extracts (vanilla, almond, etc.)
> Fruit or vegetable garnishes (a few slices of onion,
>   tomato, orange, etc.)
> Dill pickle (one pickle; high in salt)

Pickle relish (1 tablespoon; high in salt)
Salsa made without oil (3 tablespoons; may be high in salt)
Catsup (1 tablespoon; high in salt)
Barbecue sauce (1 tablespoon; high in salt)
Butter-flavored sprinkles (2 tablespoons)

VERY LOW-CALORIE RAW VEGETABLES

Lettuce	Radish
Spinach	Mushrooms
Cabbage	Celery
Sprouts	Jicama
Cucumber	Green pepper

VEGETABLES: THE SAFETY VALVE

When you're really hungry and need to supplement a meal or have a snack, reach for vegetables—especially the ones on the Next-to-Nothing list. They'll fill you up and satisfy the need to chew, while providing extra nutrients.

- ◆ Snack on crunchy raw veggies—celery, jicama, cucumber.
- ◆ Enlarge a meal with a generous serving of salad.
- ◆ Use vegetables to add bulk to sandwiches, soups, casseroles, stir fries, and other dishes.

SUGAR-FREE SWEETS

Sugar-free hard candy or gum (limit to 5 pieces)
Sugar-free gelatin dessert (limit to ½ cup, prepared)

BAKING AND COOKING INGREDIENTS

Cocoa, unsweetened (up to 1 tablespoon)
Cornstarch, flour, farina (up to 1 tablespoon)
Gelatin, dry unsweetened (up to 1 envelope)

THE PORTION PRIMER

One key to success in this plan is correct portion size. Have you ever wondered how most French women stay slim, despite the rich cream sauces and buttery pastries? Their secret is small servings. I recently attended an international nutrition conference in Paris, and went out for dinner with several French friends. By American standards, the servings were tiny. My main dish consisted of one small lamb chop, four slices of potato, and one-third cup of slivered carrots; dessert was about two tablespoons of intensely flavored lemon sorbet, served in a beautiful crystal glass. But these were just two courses in a six-course dinner. Because the servings were so small, I was able to sample a wide variety of foods—and afterward I felt satisfied instead of uncomfortably stuffed. Back in the United States, restaurant servings are three times as large! We often dish out overly large servings at home too.

Almost always, if a woman tells me she's following the food plan and not losing weight, the culprit is portion size. She may not realize that her breakfast bagel is the equivalent of three or four Grain portions, or that her normal serving of frozen yogurt is two Dairy portions.

If you're following the plan and getting the results you want, you're probably using proper portions. But if you run into trouble, I urge you to spend a day or two familiarizing yourself with correct portion size. You'll quickly learn how to estimate portions, and afterward you won't need to weigh and measure. Here are a few tips:

- ◆ Use measuring cups to serve foods like rice, pasta, mashed potatoes, and soup.

- ◆ Fill a serving utensil with water, then measure to see how much it holds. For instance, I know that my ice cream scoop holds a quarter-cup, and that my soup ladle holds a half-cup.

- ◆ Notice how a portion looks in a bowl or on your plate. Thereafter you'll recognize one cup of soup or a cup and a half of pasta.

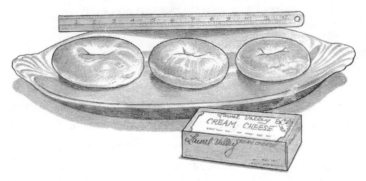

Large bagel: 4½ ounces

Medium bagel: 3½ ounces

Small bagel: 2 ounces

Bagels and other bakery items often are larger than you might expect. In the beginning, I suggest you weigh the foods you use regularly to learn how many portions they contain—remember that one ounce equals one Grain. After a while, you'll become familiar with different sizes and you'll be able to estimate.

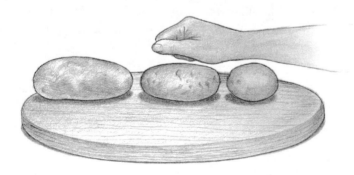

Large potato: 6 portions

Medium potato: 4 portions

Small potato: 2 portions

One Vegetable portion is just half of a small potato. A small potato is about half the size of my fist.

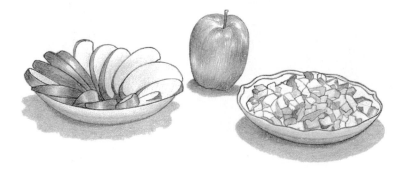

All three of the servings above contain one portion of apple. It's interesting to see that when you dice or slice an apple, it looks as though there's more to eat.

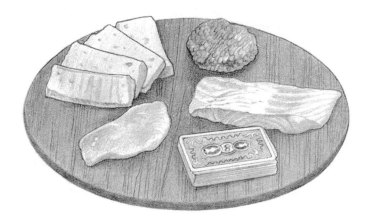

Chicken: 4 ounces

Sliced tofu: 8 ounces

Hamburger patty: 4 ounces

Codfish: 8 ounces

All of these servings are four Protein portions. Note that you get twice as much food if you eat fish or tofu. I've placed a deck of cards on the platter for reference, to help you learn how to estimate portions.

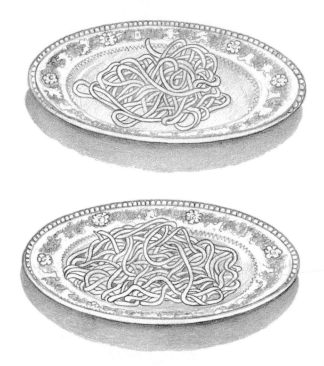

Most people don't realize how easy it is to have more pasta portions than they intend. The small serving is a half cup of cooked spaghetti, which is one Grain portion. The larger serving is twice as big—one cup, or two Grains.

SAMPLE MENUS

When I work with a woman who's beginning to follow the food plan, we start by planning menus—meals and snacks—for one or two days. I ask her to write down her favorite foods, so we can make sure they're included. We also discuss any special circumstances that affect her food choices, such as her work schedule. I encourage you to do the same. Sit down with the book and a pad, and come up with a few menus. Most women find the planning process very helpful. They're delighted to see how easily the food plan fits into their life, and they're surprised at how much they can eat.

What follows are four different menus, designed for four different women. As you'll see, their individual needs are readily accommodated. After you've been following the food plan for a while, you might welcome still more flexibility. In Chapter 12, I provide additional suggestions for specific situations.

◆　◆　◆

I lost the ten pounds I wanted to lose, and I've kept it off for a year—but I still fill out my food chart every morning and plan my three meals. It helps me stay balanced. I decide what my extras will be—wine with dinner, or candy if that's what I'm craving. If I'm going out for an Italian dinner, I plan a breakfast and lunch without Grains so I can have a big serving of pasta at night. Being organized about what I'm eating is half the battle.
　　　—Susan

◆　◆　◆

"I'M VERY BUSY; I DON'T HAVE TIME TO FUSS"

This menu is for a working mom who likes to keep things simple in the morning. It includes a brown-bag lunch and snacks for coffee breaks. A stir-fry made from salad bar vegetables provides the basis for a quick and easy dinner.

1200	1600	2000
Breakfast	**Breakfast**	**Breakfast**
Orange juice, 6 oz (1F)	Orange juice, 6 oz (1F)	Orange juice, 6 oz (1F)
Cold cereal, 1 cup (1G)	Cold cereal, 1 cup (1G)	Cold cereal, 1 cup (1G)
Skim milk, 1 cup (1D)	Skim milk, 1 cup (1D)	Skim milk, 1 cup (1D)
Sugar, 2 tsp (1E)	Sugar, 2 tsp (1E)	Sugar, 2 tsp (1E)
Snack	**Snack**	**Snack**
Cookie, 1 small (1E)	Cookie, 1 small (1E)	Cookie, 1 small (1E)
Coffee, black	Coffee, black	Coffee, black
Lunch	**Lunch**	**Lunch**
Turkey sandwich:	Turkey-cheese sandwich:	Turkey-cheese sandwich:
Lean turkey ham, 2 oz (2P)	Lean turkey ham, 3 oz (3P)	Lean turkey ham, 4 oz (4P)
1 roll, 2 oz (2G)	Low-fat cheese, 1 oz (1D, 1E)	Low-fat cheese, 1 oz (1D, 1E)
Mustard, lettuce, tomato slice	1 roll, 2 oz (2G)	1 roll, 2 oz (2G)
Baby carrots, 6 (1V)	Mustard, lettuce, tomato slice	Mustard, lettuce, tomato slice
Diet cola	Baby carrots, 6 (1V)	Baby carrots, 12 (2V)
	Raisins, 2 tbsp (1F)	Raisins, 4 tbsp (2F)
	Diet cola	Diet cola
Snack	**Snack**	**Snack**
Pretzels, 1 oz (1G)	Pretzels, 1 oz (1G)	Pretzels, 2 oz (2G)
Herb tea	Herb tea	Herb tea

1200

Dinner

Salad bar shrimp stir fry:

Oil, 2 tsp (2E)

Mixed vegetables,
1 cup (2V)

Frozen shrimp, 4 oz
(2P)

Rice, 1/2 cup (1G)

Non-fat yogurt,
1/2 cup (1D)

Frozen berries,
1/2 cup (1F)

Totals

Dairy: 2

Protein: 4

Grain: 5

Vegetable: 3

Fruit: 2

Extras: 4

1600

Dinner

Salad bar shrimp stir fry:

Oil, 3 tsp (3E)

Mixed vegetables,
1 1/2 cups (3V)

Frozen shrimp, 4 oz
(2P)

Rice, 1 cup (2G)

Non-fat yogurt,
1/2 cup (1D)

Frozen berries,
1/2 cup (1F)

Totals

Dairy: 3

Protein: 5

Grain: 6

Vegetable: 4

Fruit: 3

Extras: 6

2000

Dinner

Salad bar shrimp stir fry:

Oil, 3 tsp (3E)

Mixed vegetables,
1 1/2 cups (3V)

Frozen shrimp, 4 oz
(2P)

Rice, 1 1/2 cups (3G)

Non-fat yogurt, 1/2 cup
(1D)

Frozen berries, 1/2 cup
(1F)

Whipped cream, 2 tbs
(2E)

Totals

Dairy: 3

Protein: 6

Grain: 8

Vegetable: 5

Fruit: 4

Extras: 8

"I'M ALWAYS HUNGRY"

Appetite-appeasing features of this menu include three between-meal snacks, high-fiber choices, and items from the Next-to-Nothing list to round out meals.

1200	1600	2000
Breakfast	**Breakfast**	**Breakfast**
Orange, cut-up (1F)	Orange, cut-up (1F)	Orange, cut-up (1F)
Oatmeal, 1/2 cup (1G)	Oatmeal, 1/2 cup (1G)	Oatmeal, 1 cup (2G)
Brown sugar, 1 tsp (1/2E)	Brown sugar, 2 tsp (1E)	Brown sugar, 4 tsp (2E)
Café au lait (1/2D)	Café au lait (1/2D)	Café au lait (1/2D)
Snack	**Snack**	**Snack**
Cold cereal, 1 cup (1G)	Cold cereal, 1 cup (1G)	Cold cereal, 1 cup (1G)
Milk, non-fat, 1/2 cup (1/2 D)	Milk, non-fat, 1/2 cup (1/2 D)	Milk, non-fat, 1/2 cup (1/2 D)
Lunch	**Lunch**	**Lunch**
Broth, 1 cup (NTN)	Broth, 1 cup (NTN)	Broth, 1 cup (NTN)
Bean salad in pita:	Bean salad in pita:	Bean salad in pita:
Pita, 1 small (1G)	Pitas, 2 small (2G)	Pitas, 2 small (2G)
Chickpeas, 1/2 cup (1P)	Chickpeas, 1 cup (2P)	Chickpeas, 1 cup (2P)
Tomato, onion, salsa (NTN)	Tomato, onion, salsa (NTN)	Tomato, onion, salsa (NTN)
Fruit-flavored herbal tea	Melon, 1 cup (1F)	Melon, 2 cups (2F)
	Fruit-flavored herbal tea	Fruit-flavored herbal tea
Snack	**Snack**	**Snack**
Veggie munchies:	Veggie munchies:	Veggie munchies:
Pepper strips, mushrooms, radishes, celery sticks (NTN)	Pepper strips, mushrooms, radishes, celery sticks (NTN)	Pepper strips, mushrooms, radishes, celery sticks (NTN)
Popcorn, 3 cups air-popped (1G)	Popcorn, 3 cups air-popped (1G)	Popcorn, 6 cups air-popped (2G)
Seltzer with lime	Seltzer with lime	Seltzer with lime

1200	**1600**	**2000**
Dinner	**Dinner**	**Dinner**
Salad:	Salad:	Salad:
Lettuce, sprouts (NTN)	Lettuce, sprouts (NTN)	Lettuce, sprouts (NTN)
Low-fat dressing, 2 tsp ($1/2$E)	Low-fat dressing, 4 tsp (1E)	Low-fat dressing, 4 tsp (1E)
Garlic toast (1G, 1E)	Garlic toast (1G, 1E)	Garlic toast (1G, 1E)
Flounder, 6 oz (3P)	Flounder, 6 oz (3P)	Flounder, 8 oz (4P)
Potato, small (2V)	Potato, small (2V)	Potato, medium (3V)
Butter, 1 tsp (1E)	Butter, 1 tsp (1E)	Butter, 2 tsp (2E)
Broccoli, $1/2$ cup (1V)	Broccoli, 1 cup (2V)	Broccoli, 1 cup (2V)
Apple slices (1F)	Apple slices (1F)	Apple slices (1F)
Indian spice tea	Indian spice tea	Indian spice tea
Snack	**Snack**	**Snack**
Frozen yogurt, $1/2$ cup (1D, 1E)	Frozen yogurt, 1 cup (2D, 2E)	Frozen yogurt, 1 cup (2D, 2E)
Totals	**Totals**	**Totals**
Dairy: 2	Dairy: 3	Dairy: 3
Protein: 4	Protein: 5	Protein: 6
Grain: 5	Grain: 6	Grain: 8
Vegetable: 3	Vegetable: 4	Vegetable: 5
Fruit: 2	Fruit: 3	Fruit: 4
Extras: 4	Extras: 6	Extras: 8

"I CRAVE SWEETS"

Judicious use of Extras helps satisfy a sweet tooth. And this menu includes generous mid-day snacks.

1200	1600	2000
Breakfast	**Breakfast**	**Breakfast**
Cheese "Danish":	Cheese "Danish":	Cheese "Danish":
Cinnamon bread, toasted (1G)	Cinnamon bread, toasted (1G)	Cinnamon bread, toasted (2G)
Ricotta, non-fat, 2 oz (1D)	Ricotta, non-fat, 4 oz (2D)	Ricotta, non-fat, 4 oz (2D)
Strawberries, 1 cup (1F)	Strawberries, 1 cup (1F)	Strawberries, 1 cup (1F)
Coffee	Coffee	Coffee
Snack	**Snack**	**Snack**
Cereal, lightly sweet (1G, 1E)	Cereal, lightly sweet (1G, 1E)	Cereal, lightly sweet (2G, 2E)
Herbal tea, fruit flavor	Herbal tea, fruit flavor	Raisins, 2 tbsp (1F)
		Herbal tea, fruit flavor
Lunch	**Lunch**	**Lunch**
Hummus sandwich:	Hummus sandwich:	Hummus sandwich:
Whole grain bread (2G)	Whole grain bread (2G)	Whole grain bread (2G)
Hummus, 2 tbsp (1P)	Hummus, 2 tbsp (1P)	Hummus, 4 tbsp (2P)
Lettuce, tomato slice (NTN)	Lettuce, tomato slice (NTN)	Lettuce, tomato slice (NTN)
Carrot sticks (1V)	Carrot sticks (1V)	Carrot sticks (2V)
Seltzer with lime	Seltzer with lime	Seltzer with lime
Grapefruit, 1/2 (1F)	Grapefruit, 1/2 (1F)	Grapefruit, 1/2 (1F)
Brown sugar, 2 tsp (1E)	Brown sugar, 2 tsp (1E)	Brown sugar, 2 tsp (1E)
Snack	**Snack**	**Snack**
Chocolate milk shake:	Chocolate milk shake:	Chocolate milk shake:
Milk, non-fat, 1 cup (1D)	Milk, non-fat, 1 cup (1D)	Milk, non-fat, 1 cup (1D)
Chocolate syrup, 2 tsp (1E)	Chocolate syrup, 4 tsp (2E)	Chocolate syrup, 4 tsp (2E)
Ice cubes	Ice cubes	Ice cubes
		Animal crackers, 7 (1E)

1200	1600	2000

Dinner

Baked tortilla chips (1G)

Raw veggies (NTN)

Salsa (NTN)

Chicken breast, 3 oz (3P)

Small sweet potato (2V)

Spinach (NTN)

Decaf espresso

Midget candy bar, frozen (1E)

Dinner

Baked tortilla chips (2G)

Raw veggies (NTN)

Salsa (NTN)

Chicken breast, 4 oz (4P)

Medium sweet potato (3V)

Spinach (NTN)

Decaf espresso

Midget candy bar, 2 frozen (2E)

Apple (1F)

Dinner

Baked tortilla chips (2G)

Raw veggies (NTN)

Salsa (NTN)

Chicken breast, 4 oz (4P)

Medium sweet potato (3V)

Spinach (NTN)

Decaf espresso

Midget candy bar, 2 frozen (2E)

Apple (1F)

Totals

Dairy: 2

Protein: 4

Grain: 5

Vegetable: 3

Fruit: 2

Extras: 4

Totals

Dairy: 3

Protein: 5

Grain: 6

Vegetable: 4

Fruit: 3

Extras: 6

Totals

Dairy: 3

Protein: 6

Grain: 8

Vegetable: 5

Fruit: 4

Extras: 8

"I'M A VEGETARIAN"

Only the Protein category contains meat, and vegetarians can select from a wide variety—eggs, beans, tofu, and nuts—on this food plan.

1200	1600	2000
Breakfast	**Breakfast**	**Breakfast**
Hot wheat cereal, ¹/2 cup (1G)	Hot wheat cereal, ¹/2 cup (1G)	Hot wheat cereal, 1 cup (2G)
Skim milk, 1 cup (1D)	Skim milk, 1 cup (1D)	Skim milk, 1 cup (1D)
Banana, sliced (1F)	Banana, sliced (1F)	Banana, sliced (1F)
Coffee	Raisins, 2 tbsp (1F)	Raisins, 2 tbsp (1F)
	Coffee	Coffee
Snack	**Snack**	**Snack**
Granny Smith apple (1F)	Granny Smith apple (1F)	Granny Smith apple (1F)
		Whole wheat toast, 1 slice (1G)
		Peanut butter, 1 tbsp (1P, 2E)
		Iced tea with lemon
Lunch	**Lunch**	**Lunch**
Veggie burger sandwich:	Veggie burger sandwich:	Veggie burger sandwich:
Veggie burger, 4 oz (2P)	Veggie burger, 4 oz (2P)	Veggie burger, 4 oz (2P)
Multigrain bun, 2 oz (2G)	Multigrain bun, 2 oz (2G)	Multigrain bun, 2 oz (2G)
Lettuce, tomato, onion	Cheddar cheese, 1 oz (1D, 1E)	Cheddar cheese, 1 oz (1D, 1E)
Spicy mustard	Lettuce, tomato, onion	Lettuce, tomato, onion
Baby carrots, 6 (1V)	Spicy mustard	Spicy mustard
Club soda with lemon	Baby carrots, 12 (2V)	Baby carrots, 12 (2V)
	Club soda with lemon	Tomato juice, 6 oz (1V)
Snack	**Snack**	**Snack**
Non-fat peach yogurt, 1 cup (1D, 1E)	Non-fat peach yogurt, 1 cup (1D, 1E)	Non-fat peach yogurt, 1 cup (1D, 1E)

1200	1600	2000
Dinner	**Dinner**	**Dinner**
Grilled firm tofu, 4 oz (2P)	Grilled firm tofu, 6 oz (3P)	Grilled firm tofu, 6 oz (3P)
Grilled vegetables, 1 cup (2V)	Grilled vegetables, 1 cup (2V)	Grilled vegetables, 1 cup (2V)
prepared with:	prepared with:	prepared with:
Oil, 2 tsp (2E)	Oil, 2 tsp (2E)	Oil, 2 tsp (2E)
Teriyaki sauce, garlic, ginger	Teriyaki sauce, garlic, ginger	Teriyaki sauce, garlic, ginger
Brown rice, 1 cup (2G)	Brown rice, 1 1/2 cups (3G)	Brown rice, 1 1/2 cups (3G)
Herbal tea	Herbal tea	Herbal tea
Graham crackers, 3 (1E)	Graham crackers, 6 (2E)	Graham crackers, 6 (2E)
		Sliced strawberries, 1 cup (1F)
Totals	**Totals**	**Totals**
Dairy: 2	Dairy: 3	Dairy: 3
Protein: 4	Protein: 5	Protein: 6
Grain: 5	Grain: 6	Grain: 8
Vegetable: 3	Vegetable: 4	Vegetable: 5
Fruit: 2	Fruit: 3	Fruit: 4
Extras: 4	Extras: 6	Extras: 8

PULLING IT ALL TOGETHER

When I'm following an exercise schedule, when I'm aware of what I'm eating and how much, I feel more in control, more confident, more powerful. And that creates a ripple effect in my life. I have more patience, I'm calmer, I'm more compassionate. When my eating is out of control and when I'm not doing any exercise, I feel that other aspects of my life are out of control.
   —Therese

◆　　◆　　◆

Each component of the *Strong Women Stay Slim* weight-loss program—the strength-training exercises, the aerobic activities, and the food plan—is beneficial by itself. But they're also connected. As you bring the pieces together, you'll be pleased to discover how much they complement each other. Your aerobic workouts become easier as you get stronger. Exercise, in turn, can help regulate your appetite. And a better diet gives you more energy for physical activity. Most important, as you make healthy changes for yourself and begin to see the resulting improvements, you'll have a wonderful sense of accomplishment that will make all your efforts easier.

   Here's how to make it happen:

THE WEEK BEFORE YOU START

You've read Chapters 7, 8, and 9, which tell you how to do this program, and you may be well on your way. Perhaps you've bought dumbbells, picked out an aerobic activity, and started to plan menus. If so, congratulations! But if you need a little help to get moving, I'd like to give you some suggestions:

SIT DOWN WITH THIS BOOK, A PAD, A PENCIL, AND YOUR CALENDAR

As you know by now, I'm a strong believer in the power of lists and appointments. Just writing things down helps you get organized. Then, as you start checking off items, the list becomes both stimulus and reward. If your life is crowded with obligations, putting a task on your calendar assures uninterrupted time to get it done.

I realize that some women don't like "to do" lists and appointment calendars. If you're among them, I recommend you give yourself a deadline for starting the program. Later, if you find that the deadline has passed but you still haven't gotten moving, please give this technique a try.

GET READY TO STRENGTH TRAIN

The strength-training program requires dumbbells. If you don't have them already, reread pages 108–109 to learn what you'll need. Figure out how

IF YOU SET A STARTING DATE

You may have seen the humorous T-shirt slogan: *Eat, drink, and be merry, for tomorrow you diet.* But it's no joke when a woman overeats for five days in anticipation of starving to lose weight—and winds up feeling bloated and disgusted with herself.

Remember that there are no forbidden foods on this program. There's no need to eat a desperate "last meal." If you don't want to begin right away, give yourself a positive head start by eating more fruits, vegetables, and whole grains.

HOW TO FIND A GYM

Check your Yellow Pages under "Health Clubs" or "Exercise and Physical Fitness Programs." There may be gyms at your local community center or Y, or at a nearby school or college. Convenience is a must. You'll find it much easier to go regularly if the facility is near your home or work and the hours match yours.

Call the clubs you're considering, and arrange for a tour. If possible, visit at the same time you'd be there to work out. Here are things to look for and questions to ask:

- Is everything well lit and clean? (Use your nose as well as your eyes.)
- Do they have the kind of equipment you want to use? Is the equipment available—or are there long lines and sign-up sheets for popular machines? Are machines in good repair, or do you see many "Out of Order" signs?
- If you'd like to take classes, do they have the ones you want?
- Is the atmosphere right for you? Will you feel comfortable with the other people there? Is the sound level acceptable?
- How long has the facility been in business? Does it belong to a trade organization, such as the International Health, Racquet & Sports Club Association? Do the professional staff members have certification from reputable organizations, such as the American College of Sports Medicine or the National Strength and Conditioning Association?
- What is the fee? When comparing prices, be sure to include the extras—such as private sessions with a trainer, a permanent locker, towel service, or parking.

The International Health, Racquet & Sports Club Association (IHRSA) will send you a free brochure, *How to Choose a Quality Club*. Mail a request with a stamped, self-addressed business-size envelope to IHRSA, 263 Summer Street, Boston, MA 02210.

to get this equipment. Maybe you can share with a friend. If you're going to buy dumbbells, find a local store (check the Yellow Pages under "Sporting Goods"), or pick a mail-order source. Then make the purchase.

CHOOSE AN AEROBIC ACTIVITY

Though you won't begin aerobic exercise until the third week, start thinking about what you want to do and how you're going to get started. Do you need to buy shoes or workout clothes? A stopwatch? Other equipment? If you're planning to take the walking test, find a measured track.

Are you thinking about joining a gym? If so, have a look at the box on the previous page, which will help you select one.

♦　♦　♦

I knew I'd like working out on machines, but the idea of joining a gym was intimidating. Would a fat, middle-aged woman feel welcome? It turns out that the real *elite at my gym aren't the members with perfect bodies, but the people who show up all the time. One day about a month after I joined, the adorable little fitness instructor who was checking me in—a young woman who was literally half my age and half my size—looked at my attendance record and said, "Wow—you're really happenin' here!"*
—Sarah

♦　♦　♦

PREPARE FOR THE FOOD PLAN

You'll be exercising just three to six times weekly. But you'll be eating twenty-one times a week—and more, if you also count snacks. So planning is really important.

Reread Chapter 9 and decide which food plan to follow the first week. Come up with ideas for meals: practical breakfasts for weekdays; lunches you can take to work; dinners your family will enjoy. Think about snacks too: a pick-me-up for your coffee break; something for a long car ride; a quick bite to hold you when you come home hungry and have to prepare dinner. Look at Section IV, which has excellent, practical recipes. A well-stocked pantry will be a big help, so make a shopping list (see box, next page).

Shopping List

Vegetables
- [ ] potato
- [ ] sweet potato
- [ ] squash
- [ ] celery
- [ ] onion
- [ ] carrot
- [ ] mushroom
- [ ] broccoli
- [ ] cauliflower
- [ ] spinach
- [ ] green beans
- [ ] peas
- [ ] eggplant
- [ ] jicama
- [ ] cabbage
- [ ] lettuce
- [ ] pepper
- [ ] cucumber
- [ ] tomato
- [ ] radish
- [ ] scallion
- [ ] dill, parsley
- [ ] basil
- [ ] other herbs
- [ ] garlic
- [ ] special in-season vegetables
- [ ] canned tomato
- [ ] tomato sauce
- [ ] vegetable juice

Fruits and Juices
- [ ] orange
- [ ] grapefruit
- [ ] lemon, lime
- [ ] apple
- [ ] pear
- [ ] peach
- [ ] plum
- [ ] banana
- [ ] melon
- [ ] pineapple
- [ ] mango
- [ ] strawberries
- [ ] blueberries
- [ ] raisins; dried fruit
- [ ] special in-season fruit
- [ ] fruit juice

Dairy
- [ ] milk; buttermilk
- [ ] yogurt
- [ ] cottage cheese; ricotta
- [ ] hard cheese
- [ ] butter
- [ ] non-fat sour cream
- [ ] frozen yogurt

Proteins
- [ ] fish, seafood
- [ ] chicken, turkey
- [ ] steak, lamb
- [ ] deli meats
- [ ] eggs
- [ ] tofu
- [ ] beans—dry, canned

Grains
- [ ] bread
- [ ] pasta
- [ ] rice
- [ ] couscous
- [ ] barley
- [ ] buckwheat groats
- [ ] oatmeal
- [ ] farina
- [ ] cold cereal

Other Groceries
- [ ] pretzels, popcorn
- [ ] spices
- [ ] salsa
- [ ] balsamic vinegar
- [ ] oil, oil spray
- [ ] broth
- [ ] cocoa powder
- [ ] dry non-fat milk

Other Beverages
- [ ] coffee, tea, herbal tea
- [ ] seltzer

◆ ◆ ◆

Planning is how I protect myself from those crazy moments when I'm ravenous and standing in front of the open refrigerator, incapable of making sensible decisions about food. The bag of baby carrots is right there. It's like giving myself a willpower transplant.
—*Alexandra*

◆ ◆ ◆

PLAN YOUR ROUTINE

Now that you've figured out *how*, decide *when*. On which days will you do the strength-training exercises? What about the aerobic activity? Are you going to work out with a friend? If so, make an appointment. What's the best time for you to exercise? Early in the morning? During your lunch break? Before dinner? In the evening?

To the extent possible, create habits and routines for exercise. I realize that a weekly exercise schedule might sound like excessive regimentation, but it's actually very liberating. If you know you're doing strength training while you watch the morning news every Monday, Wednesday, and Friday, you never have to think about it.

Planning is especially important in the beginning. But it will continue to be helpful, even after you've lost weight. I strongly recommend that you set aside ten minutes at the start of each week to plan your exercise and meals. You'll be amazed at how much time you save, and how much easier the program is to follow.

SET UP YOUR LOGS

I've learned from our research projects that record-keeping really helps women follow the program correctly and remain motivated. Our volunteers agree—even those who weren't convinced at first. In fact, my assistant and I still receive logs from women who finished our studies several years ago.

Make at least ten copies of the exercise and nutrition log forms on pages 215–216 and place them in a folder or notebook. Each form covers a week. I've designed these forms to make record keeping as easy as possible— I'd much rather you spend time exercising than sitting and writing about it.

FOR THE EXERCISE LOGS

On the strength-training log, fill in the dates of each session, and list the weight of the dumbbell or the level for each exercise. Then the next time you won't have a problem remembering all the specifics. Also write down your aerobic exercise: what you did and how many minutes you spent. If you're normally sedentary, you also might want to record your Level 2 activity—remember, the more active you are, the more calories you will burn. (See pages 154–155 for a discussion of aerobic exercise intensity levels.)

FOR THE NUTRITION LOGS

At the beginning of the week, select your food plan—1200, 1600, or 2000 calories—and fill in the top row with the number of portions in each category. (This information is found in the table on page 184.) Then simply make check marks across the row in the relevant box to keep track of what you eat each day. Some women record the portions after each meal; others prefer to fill in the row at the end of the day. I've included space for notes. You might want to jot down a new food or recipe you liked, or keep track of your feelings, or record a special problem or triumph, like successfully managing a holiday dinner. These notes will be very helpful when problems come up and you're trying to devise coping strategies. Later you'll enjoy looking back to reflect on your progress.

TROUBLESHOOTING

Still having difficulty taking that first step? You're not alone. Here are the two start-up issues I hear most often—and my suggestions.

"THIS IS NOT A GOOD TIME FOR ME TO BEGIN A WEIGHT-LOSS PROGRAM"

Tomorrow night you're having twelve guests for dinner. Or you're about to set off on a two-week vacation. Maybe your dad is in the hospital, and between visits you're scrambling to keep up with your job and kids. So you're absolutely right: this is *not* the best time to start a diet and exercise program! But let's face it. If you wait for the perfect opportunity—that moment

WEEK _____ Date:_____

Weight (optional): _____

STRENGTH TRAINING LOG			
EXERCISES 2 sets/8 reps	DATE:	DATE:	DATE:
	Pounds or Level	Pounds or Level	Pounds or Level
CHAIR STAND			
OVERHEAD PRESS			
BENT-OVER ROW			
CALF RAISE			
SEATED FLY			
ARM CURL			
EXTRA EXERCISES			

AEROBIC EXERCISE LOG		
DAY	ACTIVITY	TIME (minutes)
MONDAY		
TUESDAY		
WEDNESDAY		
THURSDAY		
FRIDAY		
SATURDAY		
SUNDAY		

FOOD LOG

WEEK:	Dairy	Protein	Grain	Fruit	Vegs	Extra	Water
GOALS							8

SUNDAY	Dairy	Protein	Grain	Fruit	Vegs	Extra	Water

Notes:

MONDAY	Dairy	Protein	Grain	Fruit	Vegs	Extra	Water

Notes:

TUESDAY	Dairy	Protein	Grain	Fruit	Vegs	Extra	Water

Notes:

WEDNESDAY	Dairy	Protein	Grain	Fruit	Vegs	Extra	Water

Notes:

THURSDAY	Dairy	Protein	Grain	Fruit	Vegs	Extra	Water

Notes:

FRIDAY	Dairy	Protein	Grain	Fruit	Vegs	Extra	Water

Notes:

SATURDAY	Dairy	Protein	Grain	Fruit	Vegs	Extra	Water

Notes:

when you don't have pressure at work, stress at home, holidays, guests, or vacations—it may never arrive.

Life will always include challenges. If you're going to follow a *lifetime* eating and exercise program, you'll have to learn how to adapt. So you might as well start now, even if you take just a few steps.

Regina told me:

I'm going on a cruise next week and I want to have fun—I'll go on the program when I get back.

I wanted Regina to enjoy her cruise. But I knew that overindulgence could dampen her fun as much as excessive restraint. So I asked her to make five deprivation-free commitments to herself:

◆ Drink at least eight glasses of fluid daily.

◆ Eat at least five portions of fruits and vegetables every day—on a cruise, the chef will provide many attractive options.

◆ Set a modest aerobic exercise goal—for instance, to take at least one daily walk around the perimeter of the ship.

◆ Every other day, take five minutes to do the two strengthening exercises that don't require equipment: chair stands and toe stands.

◆ Keep a record—check marks on an index card will suffice—to track success at meeting these goals.

Minor as they might seem, these easy measures will help keep Regina from gaining weight on the cruise. And they'll ease the transition to the full program once she gets home.

"I CAN'T DO EVERYTHING AT ONCE"

When a woman tells me she feels overwhelmed by the program, I ask her which of the three components—strength training, aerobic exercise, or the food plan—would be easiest for her to follow. Then I encourage her to work on incorporating that part into her life. Once she does so, she usually finds that she can add the rest.

Dianne had described herself as "a reckless, chaotic eater." Here's how she got started:

> *Before I could think about losing weight, I needed to stabilize my eating. This took me a year, and it was an important first step. Then I started strength training. When I had been doing that for a month, I gradually began walking.*

HELP—I DON'T HAVE TIME FOR EXERCISE!

When your life is already packed to the limit, fitting in exercise isn't easy. But it's important to your health to find a way. Some possibilities:

◆ **Exercise while you watch TV.** Do strength training as you watch the evening news; use an exercise machine during your favorite sitcom. If there's any program you tune into regularly, make a habit of working out while you watch.

◆ **Transport yourself.** Instead of using your car or a bus or an elevator, take the opportunity for aerobic exercise.

◆ **Socialize while you work out.** Make exercise dates rather than lunch or dinner dates. This is a great way to spend time with your kids, your mate, your friends—even your parents.

◆ **Go on the installment plan.** If you simply can't find thirty consecutive minutes for exercise, divide your workouts into ten-minute segments and squeeze them in when you can. Get up a little earlier in the morning; take a pre-lunch or pre-dinner aerobic break. It all adds up.

For Alexandra, strength training was the key:

I knew I needed to lose weight, and I knew I should be exercising, but I wasn't ready for dieting or aerobics. Strength training appealed to me because it didn't involve sweating or getting down on the floor. After I'd been doing it for a few months, I joined a gym and began aerobic workouts on a treadmill. I wouldn't have felt comfortable joining a gym if I hadn't been strong. Also, around the same time, I began making significant changes in my eating habits. So everything came together eventually.

YOU'RE ON YOUR WAY!

During the first two weeks, you'll begin the food plan and the strength training. Unless you're already doing aerobic exercise (in which case, you should continue), you'll start during Week 3. During the next seven weeks, you'll be settling into the program. By the tenth week, you'll not only be trimmer, you'll also have new eating and exercise habits that will help you maintain a healthy weight and stay fit for the rest of your life.

If you're accustomed to overly stringent diets and exhausting exercise regimens, you may be skeptical as you begin. How can such a generous food plan and such a light exercise schedule make a difference? Yes, the steps are small at first. But this is a progressive program, and it will take you as far as you want to go.

STAYING ON TRACK

This is the third time I've lost a lot of weight. The other two times, I felt I had to be perfect, and I was—up to a point. Then everything fell apart completely, and I couldn't pull it back together. This time I haven't been perfect, and oddly enough that's the source of my greatest encouragement. I've seen that I can go on vacation for two weeks—and yes, I skip a couple of workouts and have a few big dinners—but as soon as I get home, I'm right back into my routine. I've returned to the program after a big party, after a week of houseguests, after an illness. So I know that nothing can stop me now.

—Alexandra

◆ ◆ ◆

Have you always found that it's a lot easier to lose weight than to stay slim? This time will be different. You're not going *on* a temporary diet that you'll go *off* the minute you reach a certain weight; you're making permanent changes in your life. New eating and exercise patterns will solidify into habits. Exercise will become a routine part of your day, just like brushing your teeth. You'll reach for the right foods automatically. As this transformation takes place, everything becomes easier and easier.

STAYING POSITIVE

When you begin a new program, everything seems novel and exciting. Your enthusiasm helps you get started; as you continue, it will keep you going. But this feeling needs to be rekindled from time to time. Here are some suggestions:

ENJOY YOUR WORKOUTS

I hope that physical activity becomes one of the great pleasures in your life, as it is in mine. Though my research is about exercise, my workdays at the laboratory are actually very sedentary. Getting outdoors for vigorous activity—hiking, swimming, horseback riding, biking, running, skiing—makes me feel good. And it's a great way to have fun with my family and friends.

If you find that you're not looking forward to exercising—or that you're even trying to find excuses to skip it—look for a way to refresh your routine. Here are some suggestions:

- **Try new moves**. Have a look at the extra strengthening exercises in Chapter 7 (or in Chapters 8, 11, and 12 of *Strong Women Stay Young*). You might want to change your program. In Chapter 8, I suggested that you start aerobic exercise with a single "daily bread" activity. But if it becomes a little stale, add variety. If you're walking, try another route, or switch to a bike occasionally. Rent an exercise video one day a week. Changing exercises makes your workouts more interesting, and also helps train different muscles.

- **Recruit a partner.** A workout buddy can really help you stick with an exercise program. Even if you can't find someone who will join you regularly, occasional companionship adds variety to your routine.

- **Create a distraction.** Use a personal stereo to listen to the radio, to recorded music, or to a book on tape. If you're exercising on a machine, you could watch a favorite TV show or a video.

BON APPETIT!

Variety is important for good nutrition, and also for enjoyment. While it's fine to enjoy the same foods every day—such as oatmeal for breakfast or warm milk at bedtime—don't let yourself get into a rut. If you find you're getting bored with your menus, try these ideas:

- **Plan for variety.** It's easier to expand your repertoire if you have all the necessary foods on hand. Even quick and easy recipes may require thinking ahead. For instance, brown rice is simple, high in fiber, and flavorful—but you can't wait until fifteen minutes before dinner to start cooking it.

- **Shake up your shopping.** Take a little extra time in the grocery store to check out foods you haven't tried before. Find a new kind of whole grain bread; buy an unfamiliar fruit or vegetable that's in season. Visit a new supermarket or specialty food store. You may discover interesting items in a produce store, a bakery, an ethnic grocery, or a health-food shop.

- **Look for new recipes.** For starters, check out Steven Raichlen's terrific menus and recipes in this book; you'll also enjoy his *High-Flavor, Low-Fat* cookbook series. I enjoy Jane Brody's cookbooks—her recipes are nutritious, practical, and delicious. My other favorite sources for new ideas are magazines: *Prevention* (which recently published an excellent cookbook called *The Healthy Cook*), *Cooking Light*, and *Eating Well*.

PAIN IS A FOUR-LETTER WORD

You shouldn't experience acute pain while you're exercising. Nor should you push yourself to a point that leaves you very uncomfortable afterward. Pain isn't going to make your workouts more beneficial—and it certainly won't help you enjoy them. True, you may have a little muscle soreness when you start exercising, especially if you've been sedentary. You'll also feel muscle fatigue at the end of a strength-training set. But any discomfort should be brief. Exercise should make you feel great.

In the Beginning

Your body may need time to adjust to increased activity. During the first few weeks of this program, or after you return to it following time away, it's normal to feel mild achiness. Discomfort can appear during a workout, or may be delayed until the next day. I don't recommend that you take a painkiller, because medication can interfere with the body's own repair mechanisms. Instead, try hot baths or massage. Stretching can help prevent the problem, and it may also make your sore muscles feel better.

As I'll explain below, pain can be a signal that you need medical attention. This doesn't necessarily mean you've been injured by exercising—more likely, you've uncovered an existing problem that was masked by inactivity.

For Strength Training

Learn the difference between "good" pain, which is simply muscle fatigue, and "bad" pain, which can signal an injury. Muscle fatigue is a dull ache that builds up slowly as you lift a weight, and vanishes within minutes after you stop. Bad pain is sharp and located in a joint rather than a muscle. It doesn't go away quickly and feels even worse during your next workout.

If you're experiencing the bad kind of pain while strength training, stop! Relieve the discomfort by elevating the joint and icing it. Next time you work out, try lighter weights or a more limited range of motion—whatever it takes to do the exercise comfortably. You can increase slowly from there. If pain remains severe, seek medical help.

For Aerobic Activity

Strength training will help you minimize discomfort and injuries during aerobic exercise. The same "good pain/bad pain" distinction applies to your aerobic workouts. **If you develop chest pain or tightness, pain down your arm, or severe shortness of breath, stop right away and call your doctor.** These could be symptoms of cardiac problems.

More commonly, women experience pain in their joints—ankles, knees, hips, elbows, or shoulders. Stop any activity that causes sharp pain.

Rest the affected area and treat it with ice. In a few days, resume the activity cautiously. See your doctor if the pain persists or gets worse.

SUCCESS ISN'T JUST MEASURED IN POUNDS

When you're working toward a goal, self-evaluation helps you succeed. Periodic checks ensure that if you go off track, you can quickly pull yourself back. Also, your progress is a potent encouragement. Don't just look at the scale: you're making many other positive changes as you create a healthier new lifestyle.

TO WEIGH OR NOT TO WEIGH?

Most health professionals encourage women who are losing weight to step on the scale regularly, but not daily. That's because your weight can vary by two or three pounds in a day because of differences in the amount of water in your body. If you're premenstrual, or if you ate salty food and drank a lot of fluid, you could gain; on a hot summer day, when you're perspiring copiously, you could lose water. These are normal, healthy variations.

In my experience, some women do just fine with daily weighing. They're prepared for variations and can focus on long-term trends. Others avoid the scale and track their progress in other ways. That's okay too. Figure out which approach works best for you.

◆ ◆ ◆

I never get on the scale anymore. If it didn't go down, my confidence would plummet, and that's not good. I look in the mirror; I go by how my clothes fit. Sometimes my husband will hug me, notice I feel a little different, and say, "Have you lost weight?"
—Therese

◆ ◆ ◆

I weigh myself every day, because I have to find out what's going on. I don't overreact to little fluctuations—there could be a lot of reasons for them.
—Nancy

♦　♦　♦

One caution if you opt for weekly weigh-ins: don't fall into the trap of crash dieting two days before, and then overeating afterward. The whole point of this program is to adopt a consistent, healthy eating pattern.

BODY COMPOSITION MEASUREMENTS

Some fitness centers attempt to track weight loss with a tape measure or with devices that claim to gauge body fat, such as infrared instruments or calipers that measure a fold of skin. Unfortunately, these are usually imprecise. In our laboratory at Tufts, we use more than ten different techniques to measure body composition, including MRIs, CAT scans, and underwater weighing. Believe me, if there were a simple, inexpensive way to do this reliably, we'd use it.

Outside the laboratory, the most accurate way to estimate how much body fat you've lost is to weigh yourself. If you want to try a tape, calipers, or other device, wait until you've lost at least ten pounds before you have yourself remeasured. Otherwise, you may not see a difference.

WATCHING YOUR WORKOUTS

Look for progress in your workouts. With strength training, change is easy to see. During the first ten weeks, the amount of weight you can lift should increase rapidly. Improvements come more slowly after that. But you can flex your biceps muscles and feel your leg muscles—and that's exciting.

You'll also see encouraging changes in your aerobic activity. In just a few weeks you should be able to work out for a longer time without getting tired. You'll probably notice that you have to move faster or otherwise increase the challenge of the activity to reach the correct intensity. That's a sign that your heart and lungs are getting stronger.

Periodically retake the walking test (pages 160–162) to measure improvements in your aerobic fitness. Also review your logs: see where you started and where you are now; compare yourself with the goals on pages 141 (strength training) and 164 (aerobic activity). Most women are very encouraged by how quickly they progress.

◆ ◆ ◆

The improvement was so dramatic and it happened so fast, I was shocked. Two months after I started strength training, I was using 16- and 20-pound dumbbells. For the first time in years, I could actually see my muscles.
  —Isabel

◆ ◆ ◆

BETTER MEDICAL REPORTS

One of the most satisfying changes that comes with fitness and weight loss is improved health. After your next checkup, compare the latest results with older findings. If your blood pressure, blood cholesterol, and blood sugar were elevated before, they probably will show improvements.

FEELING GOOD

The most important indicator of success is how you feel. Are you happier and less self-critical? Are you handling stress better? Has your sleep improved? Are you more self-confident? What changes do you see in your everyday life?

◆ ◆ ◆

I have a large garden, and I've just spent three days doing intensive gardening for the first time since I began the program. This is heavy work, like digging out weeds with a pitchfork. I definitely see a difference. I'm hardly sore; I can easily go up and down the back stairs with a three-gallon watering can. My husband is amazed.
  —Jane

◆ ◆ ◆

I park on the top floor of the garage at work, on level six. Now I can run up the stairs without feeling winded—I don't think twice about it. I used to get out of breath at level four.
—*Nancy*

♦ ♦ ♦

EVALUATING YOUR PROGRESS

About once a month, use the chart on page 228 to take inventory. See which pieces of the program are working well, and which need adjustment.

- **Green light**: You're doing great—continue!

- **Yellow light**: You should feel encouraged by the changes you've already made. But you need to do more in order to achieve your goals. Review the relevant chapters to get ideas and new inspiration. You should be in the green light category soon.

- **Red light**: The fact that you did the evaluation is a very good sign, because it means you're ready to get back on track. Do some planning and self-evaluation. What do you want to accomplish? What has worked in the past—and what hasn't worked? What do you need to do now? You may find it helpful to reread Chapter 5.

DEALING WITH TEMPORARY SETBACKS

It's almost impossible to follow a long-term diet and exercise plan without having problems from time to time. The answer isn't to avoid setbacks—that's impossible—but to make sure they're temporary.

How Are Things Going?

Program Component	Green Light	Yellow Light	Red Light
Strength training	I'm doing the exercises two or three times a week and making progress.	I do the exercises once a week, and I've improved a little.	I haven't been doing the exercises regularly.
Aerobic activity	I'm pretty much following the program, with three to five workouts a week.	I do at least one workout a week, but don't usually manage as many as three.	I haven't done the workouts for a week or more.
Food plan	I stick to the food plan nearly every day.	I stick to the food plan most of the time.	I haven't really followed the food plan for at least a week.
Weight	I've lost an average of half-a-pound to two pounds per week.	I've lost a little weight, but not as much as I hoped.	I haven't made progress.
Health and energy	I feel great!	I don't see much difference.	I actually feel worse.

"I CAN'T SEEM TO GET STARTED ON THE EXERCISE PROGRAM"

One helpful technique is to focus on your motivations. Take the time to write them down. Think about why you want to get fitter and lose weight. Are you trying to look better? Are you concerned about your health, because your mother developed diabetes when she was your age? Was your last vacation a disappointment because you didn't have the energy to keep up with your kids? Keep the list of your motivations where you can read it often. You'll be surprised by its power.

♦   ♦   ♦

I had a management job in high tech. The bright 20-year-olds who worked for me looked great, but I felt old and unattractive. It was hard for me to provide leadership, because I didn't feel that I was a desirable person to work for. Losing weight and becoming stronger gave me a whole new identity.
—Isabel

♦   ♦   ♦

"I'M DOING A LITTLE EXERCISE, BUT NOT AS MUCH AS I'D LIKE"

Maybe you've started the strength-training program, but not the aerobics (or the other way round). Or perhaps you're doing both, but less often than you want. I encourage you to continue—you've taken an important first step. Now it's time for the second.

Instead of setting yourself a goal that's a little too difficult, then feeling guilty when you fail, come up with an objective so easy that you're certain of success. Let's say you've been meaning to start strength training, but weeks have gone by and it just hasn't happened. Stop expecting to begin the entire program right away—that expectation isn't working. Instead, promise yourself that this week you'll do the two exercises that don't require equipment, the chair stands and the toe raises. Then next week, continue those exercises and buy the dumbbells. If you go that far, I bet you'll be doing the entire program a week or two later. There's nothing as motivating as setting a goal and achieving it.

"I'VE STARTED THE FOOD PLAN A COUPLE OF TIMES, BUT I CAN'T STICK WITH IT"

Starting and stopping is discouraging. It's better to follow a few aspects of the program consistently, even if you can't manage the whole thing. For instance, resolve to drink at least eight glasses of fluid a day, or promise yourself to switch to whole grain breads and cereals. Just concentrate on the changes you find possible. Once those are in place, other pieces of the program will seem much easier.

"EVERYTHING WAS GOING BEAUTIFULLY— THEN I WENT ON VACATION"

Brief interruptions won't keep you from your goal, provided you learn to recover quickly. Since interruptions are an unavoidable part of life, this is an important skill for permanent weight loss. And now you have the perfect opportunity to practice. The key is to get back on track as soon as you can— and to feel really good about that.

Dianne, one of the women who tested the program for this book, sounded very disheartened at one of our Monday meetings. She told the group, "I was at a barbecue over the weekend, and I really blew it." Someone asked her, "Exactly what did you eat?" As Dianne recited the list, she began to realize that she hadn't done as badly as she'd thought. Yes, she'd eaten too much chicken, too much cake, and too much in general, but she'd skipped the chips and taken a modest portion of potato salad. She had eaten much less than she would have a year ago. And even more important, she'd returned to her food plan the very next day. As I reminded her, "One meal is inconsequential when you think of your life as a whole."

◆ ◆ ◆

When I travel, I enjoy checking out other gyms. This usually costs between five and fifteen dollars per visit. Y members can visit other Ys; IHRSA (International Health, Racquet & Sports Club Association) has a free "passport" that entitles you to discounts at their member clubs all over the world. It's fun to go to a posh fitness center with a friend, and visit on side-by-side treadmills instead of at the dinner table.
—Sarah

◆ ◆ ◆

THE HUNGER CHECKLIST

Hunger is not only normal—it's desirable. Your body is reminding you to eat. You should feel hungry when you wake up in the morning and haven't eaten since the day before; you should feel hungry three to five hours after a meal. Unfortunately, hunger is an imperfect mechanism. It's not immediately relieved by eating, and sometimes it's confused with other feelings.

Use this hunger checklist to decode the urge to eat:

♦ **When did I last eat?** If your last meal was less than three hours ago, you probably don't need to eat again. Also, remember that it takes your body at least twenty minutes to "register" a meal; if you've just eaten, allow yourself enough time to feel full.

♦ **Have I had enough to drink?** Sometimes what feels like hunger is really thirst. You should be drinking at least eight glasses of fluid a day. If you feel hungry less than three hours after a meal, try drinking a glass of water.

♦ **Am I tired?** If you're fatigued, you may be looking for a quick pick-me-up. Try a nap instead of a snack—you'll be surprised at how refreshing a brief rest can be. If fatigue is a frequent problem, adjust your schedule so you get enough sleep.

♦ **Am I under stress?** When you're anxious or upset, eating can be a form of comfort and self-sedation. Instead, try a walk or some other exercise to cope. And make an effort to identify the underlying source of your distress.

As you lose weight, you'll learn to identify real hunger and distinguish it from these impostors. Gradually your desire for food will become more attuned to your body's true needs.

"I'M DOING EVERYTHING RIGHT, BUT I HAVEN'T LOST ANY WEIGHT!"

If you're following the program consistently, you'd think that your weight loss would be consistent too, but that's not always the case. It's perfectly normal to lose weight for a few weeks, level off for a few weeks, then start losing again. We're not sure why this happens. Some women retain water and gain weight just before their periods, then lose it afterward; they learn to expect this pattern.

Try not to be discouraged—you're doing something very positive for yourself, and probably just need to give it a little more time. Meanwhile, consider if either of these factors might account for the disappointing results:

Am I eating more than I realize?

This is usually the problem when people tell me they're following the food plan but not losing weight. Don't drop down to a lower calorie level until you check portion sizes. Take a look at pages 195–198 (the Portion Primer).

FOOD	RECORDED AS	BUT ACTUALLY	EXTRA CALORIES (APPROXIMATE)
Oatmeal for breakfast	1 cup	1½ cups	60
Whole wheat bread for sandwich at lunch—two thick slices cut from a bakery loaf	2 ounces (two 1-ounce slices)	4 ounces (each slice was 2 ounces)	120
Chicken breast	3 ounces	4 ounces	40
Apple	1 medium	1 large	30
Crackers with non-fat cheese spread (free sample at store)	Not recorded	½ Grain ½ Dairy	80
Broken pretzel pieces (nibbled as she set out pretzels in a bowl)	Not recorded	¼ Grain	20

Lillian lost ten pounds in the first twelve weeks, then hit a plateau. "I'm following the program religiously!" she told me—and her food diary showed she was. I asked her to try weighing and measuring for a few days, just in case.

Next week Lillian was back—one-and-a-half pounds lighter. She'd checked her portions with a scale and measuring cups, and had been startled to discover that she was eating more than she intended. As she listed the discrepancies, I tallied the extra calories. She hadn't counted them, but her body certainly had.

A series of minor slips—see table on previous page—added up to an extra 350 calories in a single day! As soon as Lillian trimmed portion size and included all snacks as part of her meal plan, her weight loss resumed. If this hadn't happened, I would have suggested that she switch to the next lower food plan—1200 calories instead of 1600.

Am I exercising at sufficient intensity?

If so, you should be making progress. With strength training, that means graduating to heavier weights during the first few months (progress normally slows after that). With aerobics, you should be able to increase the distance, intensity, or length of your workouts, especially in the early months.

If you aren't seeing changes, you might need to push yourself a little more, provided you can do so comfortably. Your aerobic workouts should raise a sweat. If they don't, check your pulse and review the exercise intensity scale (page 155).

What if you can't find an explanation? If you're following the 1200-calorie plan and doing the exercises but aren't losing weight, give yourself a couple of weeks. If you're still at a plateau, talk to your doctor. Medications and medical problems can cause weight gain or explain why you aren't losing weight on a sensible diet-plus-exercise program.

◆　◆　◆

Years ago I was on a 1200-calorie diet, and gaining weight. First two pounds, then the next week one pound. The third week, when the scale was up yet another pound, I went to my doctor. "I'm not surprised," she told me. "You're pregnant."
—Alexandra

◆　◆　◆

"MY FRIENDS FEEL GREAT ON THIS PROGRAM, BUT I'M DRAGGING"

You're wise to be concerned. Try to figure out what's going on. You might have to adjust the program—or the problem could lie elsewhere.

- **Are you eating enough?** If you're losing more than two pounds a week, or if you're losing less but feel hungry all the time, you may need more food. Just move up to the next higher calorie level. If you're already at 2000 calories, add more foods from the Next-to-Nothing list (pages 193–194). Also check portions to be sure you aren't giving yourself too little.

- **Are you drinking enough?** You need at least eight glasses of fluid a day—and more during the summer when it's hot.

- **Are you exercising too much?** Proper training should make you feel energized, not exhausted at the end of the day. If your muscles continue to feel sore, stiff, or fatigued after the first few weeks, you may be pushing too hard. Experiment with a lighter schedule to see if that restores

IF YOU WERE PREVIOUSLY ON A VERY LOW-CALORIE DIET . . .

Your metabolic system went into starvation mode, which is nature's way of helping you survive when your food supply is inadequate. Now your body will need several weeks to readjust. In the meantime, you may not lose weight—indeed, you might even gain a few pounds. Try to be patient. Once you start eating well and exercising, your metabolism should get back up to speed, and your weight loss should resume. Even before that, you should see other benefits: more energy and strength, less stress, better sleep. Focus on these improvements, which show that you're doing something good for yourself.

your energy—cut back on either the intensity or duration of exercise. Don't forget to take off one day per week.

- **Do you have a mild illness?** Give yourself a week to feel better. If you haven't improved by then, see your doctor. Sometimes a cold or other malady can sap your energy, even though it's not bad enough to send you to bed. Another possibility is that increased physical activity has uncovered a condition you didn't notice before, such as borderline anemia.

- **Are you under stress?** Look at what else is going on in your life. Pressures at work or at home could be affecting your energy.

AFTER THE FIRST TEN WEEKS

No matter how much weight you need to lose, the end of the tenth week is an important milestone. Take some time to think about—and enjoy—what you've accomplished: you've lost weight; you've established healthy eating habits; you've gotten stronger and fitter. These are wonderful gifts to yourself.

TO CONTINUE LOSING WEIGHT

If you've been losing half a pound to two pounds a week, just keep doing what you're doing. If your weight loss has slowed to less than half a pound per week but you're close to your goal, I suggest you continue your program and be content to progress more slowly.

Sometimes weight loss stalls when you're still far from finished. Check portion size. If that's not the answer, you'll need to decrease your caloric intake, increase your aerobic exercise, or do a little of both.

To Decrease Intake

Drop to the next lower calorie plan. You don't have to take the entire step at once. For example, if you're on the 1600-calorie plan, you can go to 1200 calories during the week, but continue eating 1600 calories on the weekends. If you're following the 1200-calorie plan already, don't go any lower. Either increase your exercise or try to adjust your expectations so that you're satisfied with slower change.

To Increase Exercise

Add Level 3 aerobic activity—but don't exceed one hour daily. Continue to take at least one day a week off to give your body a rest. Make sure you're getting plenty of Level 2 aerobic activity. The more you can do, the better.

If you want to add extra strengthening exercises, use the ones in this book or from *Strong Women Stay Young.* Don't work the same muscles two days in a row; they need time to rest and repair themselves.

ADJUST YOUR GOALS

Sometimes weight loss stops when you're still heavier than you want to be. You try cutting back on food, but skimpier rations leave you hungry. Adding aerobic exercise isn't appealing either—you're already working out five days a week, for a total of five hours. This situation calls for reassessment of your weight-loss goals.

If the issue is appearance rather than health, perhaps you should de-

THE LAST FIVE POUNDS

When you're just five pounds from your goal and nothing is happening, it's easy to feel impatient. Don't be tempted to take drastic measures—they rarely work in the long run. Continue following the program, but drop down to the next lower calorie level and increase physical activity.

What if the weight still doesn't budge? Ask yourself if you've *ever* been able to maintain a lower weight than you're at right now. If not, maybe your body is trying to tell you something. Try this: decide to live with your present weight for a month or two. Just concentrate on eating well and exercising. A few more pounds may slip away. Or you might find that you're content with your new shape.

cide to be content at your present weight. There are many other ways to improve how you look—consider what you might accomplish with different clothing, a haircut, new eyeglasses, or makeup. What if you're at a weight that puts you at risk according to the BMI chart? Maintain your good eating and exercise habits, but try to increase your Level 2 aerobic activity: cultivate an active hobby; walk more often during the day. The extra calories you burn will contribute to continuing slow weight loss.

WHEN YOU'VE REACHED THE WEIGHT YOU WANT TO MAINTAIN

I hope you're proud of yourself, because you deserve to be. You've lost weight—and lost it the right way, through healthy, positive change. For many women, this achievement signals that they can take on other challenging tasks.

What you've learned so far will be of enormous help. But there are three new areas to think about:

FINE-TUNING THE PROGRAM

To maintain your weight, you'll have to adjust your program. Here are things to consider as you add and subtract:

Strength Training

Some women enjoy strength training so much, they're not only eager to continue with three sessions per week but even want to add new exercises. That's just fine. However, when you're maintaining your weight, two sessions a week is sufficient.

Aerobic Exercise

You can continue your present exercise program, or cut back a little. But to stay fit, do at least twenty minutes of Level 3 aerobic activity three days a week. The more you exercise—and that includes Level 2 activity—the more you'll be able to eat without regaining.

Food Plan

If you want to continue exercising at your present level, you'll have to eat more to maintain your weight. Move to the next higher calorie level and see how that works. You can make the change gradually. Remain at your present level during the week and increase it only on weekends.

LISTENING TO YOUR APPETITE

During the weeks—or maybe months or years—of weight loss, you've eaten slightly less than your body needs. This has required you to tame your natural appetite. Now your appetite must perform its natural task, which is to regulate your food intake so it matches your energy expenditure. If you've been overweight for a long time, you may not trust your appetite at first. Focus on learning what hunger feels like, and how quickly your body registers satiation. With continuing success, you'll gain confidence.

♦   ♦   ♦

I'm making healthier choices just because that's what I prefer now. I went out for a buffet dinner on my birthday, and it wasn't a struggle to skip the creamy seafood sauce. I felt very good about that.
—*Ruth*

♦   ♦   ♦

SAFEGUARDING YOUR SUCCESS

Once you reach the weight you'd like to maintain, I suggest you weigh yourself periodically. It's all too easy for the pounds to creep back; this can happen slowly. Since you might not notice a change in your clothing immediately, the scale provides the best early warning.

Don't avoid weighing yourself because you're afraid you'll see a number you won't like. It's much better to confront the problem right away. And it's important to check, regardless of what else is happening in your life. The time you're most likely to gain is during change and disruption—when you switch jobs, get married or divorced, become ill, or take a vacation.

Everyone slips now and then. Don't be self-critical if that happens. Focus on all the positive things you've been able to accomplish. If you could do all this, you can certainly get back on track.

12

QUESTIONS AND

ANSWERS

You have to figure out ways to stay motivated. Since that can change, you need to take time to focus on yourself and think about what you're doing. It's easy to slip back into old routines. I find it helpful to reread things that have been motivating—that gives me a little shot in the arm.

—Dianne

◆ ◆ ◆

A s I wrote this book, I tried hard to anticipate your concerns. I hope that if any questions remain, they're answered here. Also, check the index in case you missed a detail. After you've been following the program for a few months, I suggest you glance over the book again. As you lose weight and gain experience with the exercise and food plans, different information will become relevant.

IF YOU HAVE QUESTIONS ABOUT THE STRONG WOMEN STAY SLIM PROGRAM

Q: I have a medical condition. Can I still do this program?

A: Nearly everyone can do this program, even people who have recovered from surgery—including joint replacement, hysterectomy, mastectomy, and other cancer treatment—as well as those with chronic but *stable* medical conditions, such as heart disease, diabetes, arthritis, osteoporosis, and joint problems. If you have a specific health concern, here are my recommendations:

- Each individual is unique. It's *very* important to discuss the program with your doctor before you start, so you can make any necessary adjustments in the food or exercise plan.

- Start conservatively and progress slowly. For instance, if you have problem shoulders, you can begin by doing the strengthening exercises without dumbbells; if that's comfortable, you can try 1-pound dumbbells, increasing the weights every two weeks instead of weekly.

- Pay attention to your body. Feeling good is your best indicator that you're exercising properly.

Q: I've just had a baby and I'm eager to get back to my pre-pregnancy weight. When can I start this program?

A: At your postpartum checkup—usually four to six weeks after birth—talk to your doctor about starting this program and losing weight. If you're healthy and doing well, you'll probably get an okay. You'll need to modify the food plan if you're breastfeeding, since you need extra calories. Start the exercises slowly and progress conservatively, because you're probably more out of shape than you expect. Even before your checkup, you can begin making healthy changes in your life. As soon as you feel able, take walks with your new baby. Eat plenty of vegetables, and drink at least eight glasses of fluid per day.

Q: I look fine if I'm sitting down, but I desperately need to do something about my hips. Can this program help?

A: Many people ask me how to focus weight loss on a particular part of the body. I wish it were possible! Strength training can firm specific muscles, and that makes a big difference. But it can't selectively eliminate the fat covering the muscles. The only way to get rid of fat (short of surgery) is to lose weight, and you can't target that.

The chair stands (see page 116) will tighten your buttocks and give you slimmer hips. Whole-body aerobic activity, such as walking, decreases overall body fat; weight-loss will help too. Remember that basic body shape seems to be part of our genetic heritage. Once you've reached a healthy weight and have accomplished what's possible with strength training and aerobic exercise, I hope you'll learn to love your feminine curves.

Q: Will this program eliminate my upper arm "bat wings"?

A: Strengthening exercise will tone and strengthen your arm muscles; aerobic exercise will decrease the fat layer on top of them. Many women are delighted by these changes; they tell me that their upper arms look better than they have in decades. By losing weight slowly, you give the skin of your upper arms more time to tighten up.

Q: Can my husband do this program with me?

A: Absolutely! The food plan, which is based on the Food Guide Pyramid, is designed to help everyone eat well. Men, like women, are advised to get at least thirty minutes of aerobic exercise a day. If your husband is currently sedentary, he can use the instructions in this book to gradually work up to that. Many men, including my husband, do the strength-training exercises and gain a lot of benefit from them. Because of their greater muscle mass, most men are able to start strength training with heavier weights, and they usually reach a higher level than women do. But the basic instructions are the same: how to make the moves; the number of sets and reps and the number of sessions per week; what intensity of effort to aim for; and how to progress.

FOR YOUR DOCTOR

Here are some of the studies and articles that underlie the *Strong Women Stay Slim* program.

◆ Miriam E. Nelson et al., "Effects of high-intensity strength training on multiple risk factors for osteoporotic fractures: a randomized controlled trial," *Journal of the American Medical Association* 1994, volume 272, pages 1909–1914.

◆ Douglas L. Ballor and Eric T. Poehlman, "Exercise-training enhances fat-free mass preservation during diet-induced weight loss: a meta analytical finding," *International Journal of Obesity* 1994, volume 18, number 1, pages 35–40.

◆ Ross E. Andersen et al., "Encouraging patients to become more physically active: the physician's role," *Annals of Internal Medicine* 1997, volume 127, pages 395–400.

◆ Steven N. Blair et al., "Influences of cardiorespiratory fitness and other precursors on cardiovascular disease and all-cause mortality in men and women," *Journal of the American Medical Association* 1996, volume 273, number 3, pages 205–210.

◆ Wayne W. Campbell et al., "Increased energy requirements and changes in body composition with resistance training in older adults," *American Journal of Clinical Nutrition* 1994, volume 60, pages 167–175.

◆ Mary L. Clem et al., "A descriptive study of individuals successful at long-term maintenance of substantial weight loss," *American Journal of Clinical Nutrition* 1997, volume 66, pages 239–246.

IF YOU HAVE QUESTIONS ABOUT YOUR WEIGHT

Q: Every time I try to lose weight, I get derailed by hunger. I'm thinking about trying an appetite suppressant. Some of my friends are taking Prozac; others are using herbal Fen-Phen. What would you suggest?

A: When women ask me about appetite suppressants, I urge them to try other measures first—drinking more fluids, eating more high-fiber foods (fruit, vegetables, and whole grains), and exercising more. Eating well and being physically active really help curb the appetite, and they have so many other positive effects. It's not clear that appetite suppressants really help in the long run—if they do, you might need to continue taking them for the rest of your life. And as we know from the Fen-Phen experience, there's always a risk of unexpected side effects. This is just as true of herbal substitutes as it is for conventional drugs.

Prozac and other anti-depressants are sometimes prescribed for weight loss because they affect serotonin levels in the brain. These are very powerful drugs, and should be taken only after careful discussion with a well-informed doctor.

Q: I'm bloated, so I look fatter than I am. Help!

A: Some women retain water and feel uncomfortably bloated. This can happen before your period or when you're going through menopause. Here are a few suggestions:

- ◆ Cut back on salt. Most of us don't need to limit salt, but we typically eat far more than our body needs. Cutting back can't hurt, and it might help. Limit or eliminate high-salt condiments, like pickles. Leave the salt shaker off the table—try a dash of lemon juice or a sprinkle of pepper or herbs instead.

- ◆ Do aerobic exercise. Physical activity improves the body's water regulation.

- ◆ Don't restrict fluids. When intake is reduced, your body will reduce output to match.

Q: I read an article that said it's important not to get heavier as I get older. But then I saw another article that said it's healthy to gain with age. Which is right?

A: This is a matter of continuing controversy. Some studies show that gaining one or two pounds per decade is beneficial because it reduces your risk for developing osteoporosis and becoming frail. But other studies find that the healthiest people are those who maintain the same body weight throughout their lives. Everyone agrees, however, that gaining more than ten to twenty pounds as you get older puts you at greater risk for heart disease, stroke, diabetes, osteoarthritis, and other conditions.

Q: Every year I gain weight in the fall, then lose most of it in the spring. What's going on?

A: This is a common pattern, and there are several possible explanations. During the colder and darker months of the year, we tend to spend more time indoors and become less active. At the same time we may eat a little more, especially during the holiday season. Some people are more prone to depression during the winter, which further contributes to both inactivity and increased eating. Fortunately, these changes usually are reversed in the spring, as we become more active. You can counter winter weight gain (and depression) by remaining physically active throughout the year.

IF YOU HAVE QUESTIONS ABOUT STRENGTH TRAINING OR AEROBIC EXERCISE

Q: Won't I get bulky if I lift weights?

A: No—you'll gain a lot of strength, but your muscles will be only slightly larger. When you combine strength training with aerobic exercise and weight loss, you shed body fat. Since a pound of fat takes up more space than a pound of muscle, even women who don't lose weight often drop a dress size or two.

HOW I ENCOURAGE MY CHILDREN
TO BE PHYSICALLY ACTIVE

My husband and I love sports, and we're fortunate that our three children—ages 6, 8, and 9—share this great pleasure. Much of what we do together as a family involves getting outdoors for vigorous physical activity.

Many weekends we head for Vermont and New Hampshire, where our parents live—ideal spots for family hikes. Last summer my husband and I, our two oldest children, my brother-in-law, and his two teenage daughters took a challenging eight-mile climb in the White Mountains. What a wonderful day! At the top, we enjoyed a spectacular view and feasted on wild blueberries. Our reward at the end was a swim in a magnificent emerald pool at the bottom of the mountain.

In the summer, when we're not hiking, we're usually in the water. When my son was 7, he did a mile-long swim with me along the edge of a New Hampshire lake. In the winter, we switch to skiing, both downhill and cross-country. And when the local pond freezes over, we go ice-skating.

Since our kids love the water, we joined a local indoor pool so they can swim year-round. On the evenings when I jog, my son accompanies me on his bike and we have a great time. Sometimes we run silly races in the backyard, laughing as we go around certain trees and keeping track of our time just for fun. Now that the children are getting older, we're beginning to play tennis—I think it's especially important to encourage youngsters to play sports that can last a lifetime. On rainy days, my husband and I push the living room furniture to the walls and bring out a long jump-rope. All the kids in the neighborhood love jumping rope in our living room!

Q: This book suggests two sets of eight reps for strength training, but another book I have recommends twelve reps. What's best?

A: Most experts agree that the best way to improve strength is with two or three sets of six to twelve repetitions. But no one knows just what the optimal mix of sets and reps is. I know from our research that two sets of eight reps can increase strength and build muscle and bone. Women find that this workout is practical and uses their time efficiently, which is important too.

Q: Will I perform better if I eat sports bars and drink athletic beverages?

A: These foods and drinks may help elite athletes get through tough endurance events, like the Iron Man Triathalon. But there's no evidence that they're better than ordinary drinks or food for the health and performance of the average active woman.

Q: Can my children do these exercises?

A: Aerobic and strengthening activities are great for kids, but the American Academy of Pediatrics does not recommend that children use free weights or exercise machines. That's because youngsters are more prone to injury than adults, and also are more likely to misuse equipment. Encourage your children to walk, run, jump rope, dance, swim, and play sports. To build strength, they can do the toe stands and chair stands from this book, which don't use equipment. Other appropriate strengthening exercises are sit-ups, push-ups, pull-ups, stationary jumps, and hill runs. Most important of all is to have fun, so that your kids gain a lifelong love of physical activity.

IF YOU HAVE QUESTIONS ABOUT THE FOOD PLAN

Q: I like to have a late dinner, but I've read that this interferes with weight loss. Is that true?

A: Many nutritionists speculate that this is true, based on experience with their clients—but it hasn't yet been confirmed by research. In any case, it's generally a good idea to have your last meal at least two hours before you go to bed. This enables you to digest most of your food before you get horizontal. Your gastrointestinal system works best when you're upright, because gravity helps move things along. You may have noticed that you're more likely to get heartburn if you lie down soon after a meal. Or you might have had the experience of going to bed after a big dinner, and the next morning you have the uncomfortable feeling that the meal hasn't moved very far. For these reasons it's best not to eat a heavy meal right before you go to bed.

Q: I'm a nurse, and I'm on different shifts throughout the month. Any suggestions?

A: You definitely face an extra challenge. Planning becomes even more important when your schedule changes so much. If you don't think ahead, you may be stuck with vending machine food because you're hungry in the middle of the night and that's all you can find.

To help yourself get organized, come up with a workable meal schedule for each shift. Try not to have your main meal too close to bedtime. Also, figure out when to shop. Develop a repertoire of wholesome brown bag specialties: sandwiches on whole grain bread; soups and stews that can be warmed in the microwave, if you have access to one; crispy salads; ready-to-eat fruit. Don't neglect fluids. Keep supplies of appealing drinks on hand, like herbal teas and flavored seltzers.

Q: I weigh more than 300 pounds, and even 2000 calories leaves me hungry. Can I eat more and still lose weight?

A: Perhaps. But first make sure you're eating as much satisfying food as the 2000-calorie plan allows. Select whole grains, which are high in satiating fiber. Choose tofu and fish for your protein, so you can enjoy larger portions. Take full advantage of the Next-to-Nothing list, which allows very generous quantities of filling vegetables that don't add many calories. If all this still leaves you hungry, try supplementing your daily plan with two fruits or a fruit and a vegetable.

Q: Can I use a sugar substitute?

A: You can, but I don't recommend it. First, there's not much evidence that sugar substitutes help with long-term weight control. Adding a substitute to coffee instead of sugar saves you just 14 calories, not a significant amount. Second, there are nagging questions about safety and side effects. But most important: when you use substitutes, you aren't allowing yourself to develop the healthier food preferences that will make it much easier to stay slim. Women who cut back on sugar without resorting to substitutes may feel deprived at first. But after a brief period, they almost always find that their cravings for sweet foods diminish.

Q: What about fat substitutes, like Olestra?

A: There are more than 300 different types of fat substitutes on the market, some natural and some synthetic. The natural ones are made from proteins and carbohydrates, and contain about half the calories of fat. One example is Oatrim, made from oats; it's used by some cookie manufacturers to add the texture and feel of fat. Another example is fruit puree, which can substitute for fat in some baked goods.

Olestra and other synthetic fat substitutes have no calories. They can be used to fry potato chips and other foods. If eaten in large quantities, foods made with Olestra can cause unpleasant gastrointestinal side effects. Also, even though these products are enriched with some vitamins, many nutritionists are concerned that people who use them will miss out on other valuable nutrients that require fat to be absorbed.

While all these products appear to be safe, there's no evidence that they make much of a difference for weight loss in the long run. People seem to eat larger portions of foods made with fat substitutes, which offsets the calories they save.

Q: Sometimes I have to eat at a fast-food restaurant. Can you give me any recommendations?

A: Check the menu carefully. Order fruits and salad or vegetables if possible, and select the leanest option for your main dish. Have a large glass of water or a calorie-free drink. Servings may be large—take that into account when you figure out your portions for the day. If you find you're often eating at fast-food restaurants where it's hard to follow your food plan, take some time to figure out alternatives. Maybe you can bring food from home or find other restaurants. If it's just an occasional meal, simply do your best to adapt and don't worry about it.

Q: I know I should eat three well-balanced meals, but some days I just don't have time. Is it okay to eat a meal replacement bar instead of breakfast or lunch?

A: In the long run, it's best for you to organize your day and week so you can eat real food. An occasional replacement won't do any harm—and it's certainly better than grabbing a candy bar. However, whole foods bring so much more to your diet; they're healthier and more satisfying.

Q: I don't always want all my Extras, but I'd like additional fruit or meat. Is there any way to substitute?

A: Yes. Instead of using the Extras for fats, sweets, or alcohol, you may exchange them for additional portions of the other food groups, as follows:

1 Dairy portion	= 2 Extras
1 Protein portion	= 1 Extra
1 Grain portion	= 2 Extras
2 Vegetable portions	= 1 Extra
1 Fruit portion	= 2 Extras

Q: I don't eat meat. Can I substitute dairy foods for proteins?

A: It's fine to substitute one Dairy for two Proteins, because dairy foods contain high-quality protein. Don't exchange more than two Proteins per day, because tofu, nuts, and eggs have other valuable vitamins and minerals. Since the foods in the Protein list aren't high in calcium, you can't swap in the other direction.

Q: I love potatoes, but if I eat a big potato, I use up my Vegetable portions and that doesn't seem like a good idea.

A: You're right—you need other vegetables too. What you can do is to substitute two portions of potato for a Grain. For example, a small potato, which is two Vegetable portions, can be counted as one Grain.

Q: My kids and husband won't eat this food, so I'm making different meals for everyone. It's like running a restaurant. What can I do?

A: As a mother, I can really sympathize. Fortunately, this is a very flexible food plan, so you should be able to make it work for everyone. It's also a healthy way of eating that will benefit other members of your family. Here are a few suggestions:

- Find a compromise between convenience and individual preferences. I serve one meal for dinner, but my husband and kids can have their own choices at other meals.

- Get your children (and husband) involved in meal planning and cooking.

- Encourage your kids to try new foods.

- Have very simple foods on hand—cereals, fruits, bread— when you're serving something that one family member dislikes.

Q: I'm lactose intolerant. How can I get enough calcium?

A: Dairy products contain a sugar called lactose that some people can't easily digest. Lactose intolerance could be the problem if you develop gas, cramps, or other gastrointestinal problems after consuming dairy foods. These suggestions might help:

- Have just half a portion of dairy food at a time. You may be able to tolerate small quantities without distress.

- Buy products to which lactase has been added—that's the enzyme that digests lactose. Or buy the enzyme, which comes in pill form (available in drug and health food stores), and consume it along with dairy portions.

- Select dairy foods that don't contain undigested lactose, such as cheese or yogurt made with live cultures.

◆ If the above suggestions don't work, get calcium from non-dairy sources, such as calcium-fortified orange juice or soy milk, tofu made with calcium sulfate, canned fish with bones, collard greens, broccoli, or spinach.

"I LIKE VEGETABLES, BUT I FIND IT HARD TO GET ENOUGH OF THEM"

Most of us enjoy eating vegetables a lot more than we enjoy preparing them. Here are some tips from women who've followed this food plan:

◆ Use ready-to-eat veggies for snacks, like baby carrots or broccoli flowerets.
◆ Eat vegetables in the form of soups and juice. One-portion cans of vegetable juice make great snacks for the car or office.
◆ Buy bagged, ready-to-eat lettuce to streamline salad preparation.
◆ Use salad bar vegetables, not only for salads but also for snacks, stir-fries, and cooked side dishes.
◆ Learn how to prepare vegetables quickly in the microwave.
◆ Try having vegetables at breakfast. For instance, add chopped vegetables to an omelet.
◆ Grate vegetables into soups, casseroles, meat loafs, homemade breads, and even cakes.

Q: I want to take a calcium supplement. Which kind is best?

A: The two best types are calcium carbonate and calcium citrate. Select either, but take it with 400 to 700 international units of vitamin D for greatest benefit. Calcium carbonate supplements should be taken with a meal, since the stomach acid released during digestion helps with absorption.

HOW TO COPE WITH BUFFETS AND BANQUETS

Delicious food is an important part of celebrations, holidays, and other special occasions. But temptation can be a problem. Here are some suggestions from women in the group that tested this program:

- ◆ Provide low-calorie options. If you're the hostess, make extra salads or vegetable side dishes. If you're a guest, offer to bring a fruit salad for dessert or a low-fat dip and veggies for an appetizer.
- ◆ Fill up with a bowl of vegetable soup or a salad half an hour before the party.
- ◆ Eat very, very slowly.
- ◆ Delay helping yourself at a buffet; postpone taking seconds. You'll probably eat less because you have less time; also, the food may run out.
- ◆ Cruise a buffet table before filling your plate, and take only the items you really want.
- ◆ Forget the "clean plate club"—don't eat anything you don't really enjoy.
- ◆ At a cocktail party or buffet, stand with your back to the food and talk a lot!
- ◆ Send extras home with your guests, or ask a friend to help you put them away quickly. Clean-up is often the most difficult time if you're the hostess, because it's hard to resist leftovers when you're no longer distracted by the party.

TROUBLESHOOTING

Q: I went to a brunch buffet and ate much more than I intended. What should I do about dinner?

A: The fact that you're ready to resume your food plan means that the brunch will have no long-term consequences. Don't skip dinner—that could lead to excessive hunger and more problems the next day. Just eat lightly.

Q: My friend and I started the program together six weeks ago. She's lost ten pounds but I've only lost three, and I'm getting very discouraged.

A: Please don't be unhappy—you've lost three pounds, which is terrific! You have to realize that everyone is different. If your friend is much younger or much heavier than you are, her basal metabolic rate is almost certainly higher. There may be subtle differences in her food choices, or she may be burning extra calories because she does more Level 2 activity. Try to focus on your own excellent progress: you've lost weight, and you're gaining important benefits by eating better and exercising. Stick with it, and you'll continue to lose weight.

Q: I've just gotten over the flu. How soon can I resume my workouts?

A: Don't try to lose weight while you're sick. Stop exercising and take care of yourself. Once you're over the illness—when you no longer have a fever or feel sick—start back slowly. Cut the intensity and time of your workouts in half, and see how that goes. If you feel fine, work back up to your previous level. That could take just a week or two if you had a cold, or longer if your illness was more severe.

Q: I was doing great. Then I had a family crisis and stopped exercising for nearly two months. I want to get going again, but I'm not sure where to start.

A: Your earlier success will be a great help. You already have the dumbbells; you know the strength-training moves; you've selected an aerobic activity. However, you can't expect to resume at the same point you reached before. Reduce the intensity of your exercise sessions: with strength training, drop down a level or use a weight that's half what you were lifting before. With aerobic activity, decrease the time by half (but don't do less than ten minutes). You'll quickly bounce back. In two or three weeks you'll be where you were before, and ready to progress.

FOR MORE INFORMATION

There are many very good resources for people interested in weight loss, nutrition, and exercise. If you want to learn more about how strength training affects muscles, bones, and balance, you might want to read my first book, *Strong Women Stay Young* (Bantam, 1997). Here are some of my other personal favorites:

♦ *Nutrition Navigator Web site,* presented by the Center on Nutrition Communications at the Tufts University School of Nutrition Science and Policy, is an excellent resource that has referrals to hundreds of online information sources about health and nutrition: http://navigator.tufts.edu.

♦ *Tufts University Health & Nutrition Letter* (P.O. Box 57857, Boulder, CO 80322-7857; tel. 800-274-7581 or, in Colorado, 303-447-9330.)

♦ *Shape-Up America!,* a program started by C. Everett Koop, M.D. has excellent information about fitness and weight loss. Write to Shape-Up America, 6707 Democracy Boulevard, Suite 107, Bethesda, MD 20817; or check out their Web site: http://www.shapeup.org.

♦ *ACSM Fitness Book,* by American College of Sports Medicine (Human Kinetics, 1997; P.O. Box 5076, Champaign, IL 61825-5076; tel. 800-747-4457; http://www.humankinetics.com).

- ***Biomarkers**: The 10 Determinants of Aging You Can Control*, by William Evans, Ph.D., and Irwin H. Rosenberg, M.D., with Jacqueline Thompson (Simon & Schuster, 1991).

- *The Wellness Guide to Lifelong Fitness*, by Timothy P. White, Ph.D., and the editors of the *University of California at Berkeley Wellness Letter (REBUS*, distributed by Random House, 1993).

- *The Wellness Encyclopedia of Food and Nutrition*, by Sheldon Margen, M.D., and the editors of the *University of California at Berkeley Wellness Letter* (Subscription Department, P.O. Box 44022, Palm Coast, FL 32142).

- *Human Nutrition*, by Helen A. Guthrie, Ph.D., R.D., and Mary Frances Picciano, Ph.D., (Mosby-Year Book, Inc., 1995; 11830 Westline Industrial Drive, St. Louis, MO 63146; tel. 800-426-4545; http://www.mosby.com). This is the classic basic nutrition textbook, used in Nutrition 101 at Tufts.

- *Thin for Life*, by Anne M. Fletcher, M.S., R.D. (Chapters Publishing Limited, 1994).

- *Nancy Clark's Sports Nutrition Guidebook*, by Nancy Clark, M.S., R.D. (Human Kinetics, 1996; P.O. Box 5076, Champaign, IL 61825-5076; tel. 800-747-4457; http://www.humankinetics.com).

- *Jane Brody's Good Food Book*, by Jane Brody (Bantam, 1985).

IV

MENUS AND RECIPES
BY STEVEN RAICHLEN

▼ ▼ ▼ ▼

INTRODUCTION BY MIRIAM NELSON

I love to eat good food. In the summer, I enjoy luscious ripe fruit and crispy vegetables (especially the sweet carrots that my kids pull from my brother-in-law's garden); in the winter I savor hearty soup and just-baked whole grain bread. Special dinners with family and friends are high points in my life. I'm always looking for new recipes that are wholesome but also delicious. Some of my favorites come from Steven Raichlen, author of the prize-winning *High-Flavor, Low-Fat* cookbooks. He has a special knack for creating dishes that delight the taste buds while trimming excess calories. So when I decided to include menus and recipes in this book, I turned to Steven.

I requested exciting, enticing recipes but reminded him that most of us can't spend hours in the kitchen. I wanted to expand my repertoire—I confess that I sometimes fall into a rut and wind up making the same few dishes over and over. However, I'm slightly intimidated by long lists of exotic ingredients. I asked for suggestions that could introduce variety—such as unusual fruits and vegetables, flavorful teas, and interesting spices—but without a lot of effort.

Steven was intrigued by the challenge of working within the food plan. He came up with ten remarkable menus that contain just 1200 calories for an entire day of flavor-packed eating (plus simple additions for those on the 1600- or 2000-calorie plans). I hope you'll be thrilled—as I was—to see how well you can eat on the *Strong Women* program. This is the kind of food I'd expect at a world-class health spa!

If you were a spa chef, you might follow these ten menus over the next couple of weeks, but we really don't expect you to do that. If you're like me, when you make a big casserole over the weekend, you want to coast on the leftovers during the week. And since I don't have unlimited pantry space, I tend to buy just one or two types of tea and use those up before I get another. But I hope you'll return again and again to these menus—and to the individual recipes—when you want to add zest to your meals. They're an inspiration.

This chapter proves that healthy can be delectable and that you don't have to give up wonderful food to lose weight. Bon appétit!

IN CASE YOU'RE WONDERING . . .

◆ **About snacks:** All the daily menus include meals plus snacks. Sometimes there's just one snack, sometimes there are several—and the time of day varies too. Feel free to adapt the day's allotment to your preferences. For example, you could move a morning snack to afternoon, or add an evening snack by saving dessert from lunch or dinner.

◆ **About beverages:** If a beverage isn't specified for a meal or snack, have a glass of water or another Next-to-Nothing drink. Remember, it's important to get enough fluids, both for health and for satiety.

◆ **About portions:** For menu items that are made from recipes, eat one serving and count portions as the recipe indicates. For other items, such as mashed potatoes or frozen yogurt, eat one portion (see Chapter 9 for portion sizes) unless otherwise indicated.

◆ **About exotic ingredients:** A large supermarket should have just about all the items called for in these menus and recipes. You could also try a health food store or a gourmet food shop for unusual spices, cereals, teas, fruits, types of rice, and frozen whole grain waffles.

A Vegetarian Feast

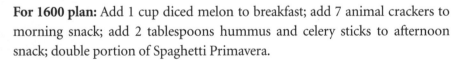

BREAKFAST

Cream of wheat cereal with blueberry syrup (p. 308)
Indian spice tea

LUNCH

Mexican bean salad with pumpkin seeds (p. 279)
Tortilla crisps (p. 275)
Club soda with lime

SNACK

1 orange

DINNER

Green salad sprinkled with balsamic vinegar
Garlic bread (p. 276)
Spaghetti primavera with grilled vegetables (p. 287)
Sliced mango

For 1600 plan: Add 1 cup diced melon to breakfast; add 7 animal crackers to morning snack; add 2 tablespoons hummus and celery sticks to afternoon snack; double portion of Spaghetti Primavera.

For 2000 plan: Add 1 cup diced melon to breakfast; add 7 animal crackers to morning snack; double portion of Tortilla Chips; add 2 tablespoons hummus and celery sticks to afternoon snack; double portion of Spaghetti Primavera; double portion of Garlic Bread; double portion of salad; add evening snack of 1 tablespoon peanut butter on sliced Granny Smith apple.

Quick and Easy

BREAKFAST
Fruit juice spritzer (p. 304)
Granola parfait (p. 308)

SNACK
Tamari popcorn (p. 275)
Club soda with lime

LUNCH
Tomato juice
Carrot sticks
Roast beef sandwich on sourdough bread
with horseradish and radish sprouts (p. 284)

DINNER
Spicy ginger turkey stir-fry (p. 294)
Brown rice
Melon salad with yogurt and mint (p. 298)
Iced green tea

SNACK
Chocolate milk
Cinnamon graham crackers

For 1200 plan: Have 1 cup brown rice at dinner.

For 1600 plan: Add extra 1 ounce roast beef to sandwich; add nectarine to lunch; add afternoon snack of 3 tablespoons of salsa, 1 ounce baked tortilla chips, and 1 ounce low-fat cheddar.

For 2000 plan: Add 2 ounces roast beef and 1 slice of bread to sandwich; add nectarine to lunch; add afternoon snack of 6 tablespoons of salsa, 2 ounces baked tortilla chips, and 1 ounce cheddar; double Melon Salad portion for dinner.

Delectably Different

BREAKFAST

Orange juice
Mexican egg scramble with toasted tortillas (p. 306)
Café de olla (p. 305)

LUNCH

Garlic grilled portobello-goat cheese sandwich
on multigrain roll (p. 285)
Iced tea with fresh mint

SNACK

Chocolate frozen low-fat yogurt

DINNER

Bulgur salad with tomato and mint (p. 277)
Fish en papillote (p. 297)
Asian pear

For 1600 plan: Double portion of Egg Scramble at breakfast; at lunch, increase goat cheese to 2 ounces and add 1 cup sliced strawberries.

For 2000 plan: Double portion of Egg Scramble at breakfast; add midmorning snack of 1 tablespoon peanut butter with celery sticks and sliced apple; at lunch, increase goat cheese to 2 ounces and add 1 cup sliced strawberries and 1 ounce pretzels; add a whole grain roll to dinner; add evening snack of hot chocolate.

A Summer Sizzler

BREAKFAST

Peach yogurt smoothie (p. 304)
Multigrain toast

SNACK

Veggie sticks

LUNCH

Gazpacho salad (p. 280)
Garlic pita chips (p. 276)
Next-to-nothing mushroom pâté (p. 273)
Iced raspberry tea

SNACK

Frozen strawberry non-fat yogurt

DINNER

Moroccan lamb kebabs (p. 293)
Lemon couscous (p. 283)
Blueberry soup (p. 300)
Mint tea

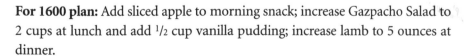

For 1600 plan: Add sliced apple to morning snack; increase Gazpacho Salad to 2 cups at lunch and add ¹/₂ cup vanilla pudding; increase lamb to 5 ounces at dinner.

For 2000 plan: Add extra slice of bread and 2 tablespoons non-fat cream cheese to breakfast; add sliced apple to morning snack and double the vegetable portion; increase Gazpacho Salad to 2 cups at lunch and add ¹/₂ cup vanilla pudding; increase lamb to 5 ounces at dinner; add evening snack of 3 tablespoons peanuts, 2 tablespoons raisins, and 1 ounce pretzels.

A Weekend Celebration

BREAKFAST

Whole grain waffles
Applesauce
Café latte (p. 306)

LUNCH

Vegetable sticks
Hungarian cheese dip (p. 274)
Vegetable juice

DINNER

Garlic soup (p. 276)
Paella Valenciana (p. 288)
Peaches in sparking wine (p. 303)

For 1600 plan: To lunch, add sandwich of 1 ounce pita, 2 tablespoons of hummus, with diced lettuce, tomato, and green pepper; add afternoon snack of lemon yogurt with 1/2 cup diced fruit.

For 2000 plan: Add extra waffle and 1/2 cup applesauce to breakfast; to lunch, add sandwich of 2 ounces pita, 4 tablespoons of hummus, with diced lettuce, tomato, and green pepper; add afternoon snack of lemon yogurt with 1/2 cup diced fruit; add 2 anise cookies at dinner.

East Meets West

BREAKFAST
Shredded wheat cereal with skim milk
Sliced pear
Apple spice tea

LUNCH
Chicken broth
Pita chips with Asian bean dip (p. 272)

SNACK
Strawberry banana low-fat yogurt

DINNER
Marinated mushroom kebabs (p. 272)
Shabu-shabu (Japanese fondue)
with lemon-ginger dipping sauce (p. 295)
Jasmine rice
Strawberry Napoleon (p. 301)

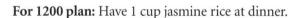

For 1200 plan: Have 1 cup jasmine rice at dinner.

For 1600 plan: Add midmorning snack of ¹/₂ cup low-fat cottage cheese and ¹/₂ cup pineapple chunks; at lunch, increase Bean Dip to 1 cup and Pita Chips to 2 portions, and add carrot sticks; add graham crackers to afternoon snack.

For 2000 plan: Add 2-ounce bagel, 2 tablespoons of low-fat cream cheese, and 2 teaspoons of jam to breakfast; add midmorning snack of ¹/₂ cup low-fat cottage cheese and ¹/₂ cup pineapple chunks; at lunch, increase Bean Dip to 1 cup and Pita Chips to 2 portions, and add carrot sticks and 2 plums; add graham crackers to afternoon snack; at dinner, double the portion of mushrooms and increase protein to 4 ounces.

Something Exotic

BREAKFAST

Puffed millet cereal with milk and sliced starfruit
Vietnamese iced coffee (p. 305)

SNACK

Slice of whole wheat cinnamon-raisin bread
Club soda with raspberry-lime flavor

LUNCH

Bulgur lettuce roll-up with spicy yogurt dipping sauce (p. 278)
Iced ginseng tea

SNACK

Indian milk shake with rose water (p. 303)

DINNER

Teriyaki salmon with spicy slaw (p. 290)
Sticky rice
Coconut fruit salad (p. 300)

For 1200 plan: Have 1 cup sticky rice at dinner.

For 1600 plan: Add slice of raisin bread to morning snack; add fresh orange and 1/2 cup frozen yogurt to lunch; for dinner, increase salmon to 5 ounces and slaw to 2 cups.

For 2000 plan: Add slice of raisin bread to morning snack; add fresh orange and 1/2 cup frozen yogurt to lunch; add dinner appetizer of 4 celery stalks stuffed with 2 tablespoons low-fat cream cheese, and increase salmon to 6 ounces and slaw to 2 cups; add evening snack of whole wheat English muffin with 2 teaspoons of honey and a banana.

Winter Warmer

BREAKFAST

Oatmeal with brown sugar
Fuji apple
English breakfast tea

LUNCH

Veggie melt on pumpernickel with tomato and jicama (p. 285)
Lemon-mint spritzer (p. 304)

SNACK

1 slice anadama bread with non-fat cream cheese

DINNER

Sliced cucumber sprinkled with fresh dill
Chicken paprikas (p. 286)
Poppy seed noodles (p. 283)
Clementine orange

LATE NIGHT COMFORT

Hot chocolate

For 1600 plan: Increase breakfast oatmeal to 1 cup made with 1 cup skim milk and 2 teaspoons of brown sugar; add 1 pear to lunch; increase dinner chicken serving by 1 ounce.

For 2000 plan: Increase breakfast oatmeal to 1 cup made with 1 cup skim milk and 2 teaspoons of brown sugar; add 1 apple and second slice of bread and cream cheese portion to afternoon snack; add 1 pear to lunch; increase chicken serving by 2 ounces and double portions of noodles and vegetables at dinner.

Vegetarian Favorites

BREAKFAST

Grits with chopped apple
Earl Grey tea

LUNCH

Greek salad sandwich (p. 284)
Mint tea with lemon

SNACK

Piña colada low-fat yogurt

DINNER

San Antonio slaw (p. 281)
Three-bean chili (p. 289)
Corn bread
Persimmon

For 1600 plan: Add midmorning snack of 1 ounce Spiced Walnuts (p. 275); at lunch, add second Greek Salad Sandwich and a navel orange.

For 2000 plan: Add midmorning snack of 2 ounces Spiced Walnuts; at lunch, add second Greek Salad Sandwich and a navel orange; add sliced banana to afternoon snack; at dinner, increase corn bread from 2 ounces to 4 ounces and add 1 cup of slaw.

A Mediterranean Celebration

BREAKFAST

Grapefruit half
Cinnamon-orange popover with jam (p. 307)
English breakfast tea

LUNCH

Fusilli salad with cherry tomatoes and arugula (p. 282)
Whole grain crackers
Tangerine with nonfat yogurt

SNACK

Broccoli florets
Garlic-yogurt dip (p. 274)

DINNER

Mixed salad with balsamic vinegar
Bouillabaisse with garlic toasts (p. 292)
Orange custard (p. 299)
Espresso

For 1600 plan: Add 2 teaspoons jam for breakfast; for midmorning snack, add sandwich made with 1 slice whole wheat bread, 1 ounce turkey, 1 ounce cheese, and 1 sliced apple; increase salad serving to 2 cups for dinner.

For 2000 plan: Add 1 popover and 2 teaspoons jam for breakfast; for midmorning snack, add sandwich made with 2 slices whole wheat bread, 2 ounces turkey, 1 ounce cheese, and 1 sliced apple; double broccoli in afternoon snack; increase salad serving to 2 cups for dinner; add evening snack of 7 animal crackers and 1/4 cup dried fruit.

APPETIZERS AND SNACKS

SALADS AND SIDE DISHES

SANDWICHES

ENTRÉES

DESSERTS

BEVERAGES

BREAKFASTS

Asian Bean Dip

The Far East meets the Middle East in this offbeat Asian twist on hummus. Serve the dip with vegetable chips, rice crackers, or toasted pita chips. Hoisin sauce, a sweet Chinese condiment made with soybeans, is available at most supermarkets.

> 1 16-ounce can chickpeas, drained, rinsed with cold water, and
>   drained again
> 1 garlic clove, minced
> 2 scallions, finely chopped
> 2 teaspoons grated fresh ginger
> $1^1/_2$ tablespoons soy sauce
> 1 tablespoon hoisin sauce (if unavailable, use 2 teaspoons
>   more soy sauce and $^1/_2$ teaspoon more sugar)
> 1 tablespoon rice vinegar or distilled white vinegar
> 2 teaspoons sugar

Combine the ingredients in a food processor and puree until smooth. Season to taste, adding soy sauce or sugar as needed.

Makes four $^1/_4$-cup servings

PER SERVING: 1 PROTEIN

Marinated Mushroom Kebabs

Mushrooms make a great Next-to-Nothing snack. This recipe is modeled on the French hors d'oeuvre *champignons à la Grecque* ("in the style of Greece").

> 4 cups mushrooms (choose small mushrooms that are all the same
>   size)
> 8 pearl onions, cut in half
> $^3/_4$ cup dry white wine
> $^3/_4$ cup vegetable or defatted chicken stock
> 3 tablespoons fresh lemon juice

1 tablespoon tomato paste
2 teaspoons ground coriander
$^1/_2$ teaspoon black pepper
1 bay leaf
Salt to taste

1. Wipe the mushrooms clean with a damp cloth and trim off the ends of the stems. In a deep saucepan, bring the onions, wine, chicken stock, lemon juice, tomato paste, coriander, pepper, and bay leaf to a boil.
2. Add the mushrooms and briskly simmer until the mushrooms and onions are tender and the cooking liquid is reduced to a thick sauce, about 15 minutes, stirring often. Add salt—and more lemon juice if needed—to taste. Transfer the mushrooms and liquid to a bowl and let cool to room temperature, then refrigerate until cold.
3. Serve the mushrooms and onions with bamboo skewers for picking them up. Or, if you like, thread the mushrooms and onions on skewers to make kebabs.

Makes four servings

PER SERVING: 1 VEGETABLE (OR NEXT-TO-NOTHING)

Next-to-Nothing Mushroom Pâté

Here's a mushroom spread that's loaded with flavor, not fat. The secret is to roast the vegetables in a hot oven to concentrate their flavor.

8 ounces button mushrooms, trimmed and quartered
$^1/_2$ small onion, peeled and cut into quarters
2 garlic cloves, peeled
1 teaspoon olive oil
Salt and freshly ground black pepper
2 tablespoons finely chopped parsley, preferably flat-leaf
2 teaspoons Cognac (optional)
1 to 2 tablespoons dried bread crumbs, or as needed

1. Preheat the oven to 450° F. Place the mushrooms, onion, and garlic in a

nonstick roasting pan. Toss with the olive oil and salt and pepper to taste. Roast the mushrooms until nicely browned, 15 to 20 minutes, stirring to ensure even cooking. Let the mushrooms cool to room temperature.

2. Puree the vegetables in a food processor, adding the parsley, Cognac, and salt and pepper to taste. If the spread seems too wet, add a tablespoon or two of bread crumbs.

Makes 1 cup or eight 1-ounce (2-tablespoon) servings

PER SERVING: NEXT-TO-NOTHING (OR 1 VEGETABLE)

Garlic-Yogurt Dip

$1/4$ cup non-fat plain yogurt
1 garlic clove, crushed
$1/4$ teaspoon grated lemon zest
Salt and freshly ground pepper

Combine the yogurt, crushed garlic, and lemon zest. Add salt and pepper to taste.

Makes one serving

PER SERVING: $1/4$ DAIRY

Hungarian Cheese Dip

1 cup non-fat cottage cheese
$1/2$ teaspoon onion powder
$1/2$ teaspoon garlic powder
$1/2$ teaspoon paprika
$1/2$ teaspoon dry mustard
Salt and freshly ground pepper

Puree the cottage cheese in a food processor with the onion powder, garlic powder, paprika, and dry mustard. Add salt and pepper to taste.

Makes two $1/2$-cup servings

PER SERVING: 1 DAIRY

Spiced Walnuts

> 3 tablespoons walnuts
> Olive oil cooking spray
> Pinch of garlic salt
> Pinch of pepper
> Pinch of paprika
> Pinch of cumin

Spray the walnuts with olive oil cooking spray. Toss with the garlic salt, pepper, paprika, and cumin.

Makes one serving

PER SERVING: 1 PROTEIN, 1 EXTRA

Tamari Popcorn

> 3 cups air-popped popcorn
> 3 tablespoons tamari (a naturally brewed soy sauce available in health food stores)

Sprinkle the popcorn with the tamari.

Makes one serving

PER SERVING: 1 GRAIN

Tortilla Crisps

> 1 flour tortilla
> Pinch of chili powder
> Pinch of garlic salt

Cut a flour tortilla into wedges and sprinkle with chili powder and garlic salt. Bake on a nonstick baking sheet in a 400° F. oven until crisp, 3 to 5 minutes.

Makes one serving

PER SERVING: 1 GRAIN

Garlic Bread

> 1-inch slice of French bread
> Olive oil cooking spray
> 1 garlic clove, minced (or ¼ teaspoon garlic powder)
> 1 teaspoon Parmesan cheese

Spray the bread with olive oil cooking spray and sprinkle with the minced garlic (or garlic powder) and Parmesan cheese. Bake in a 350° F. oven for about 10 minutes, or until crisp and golden brown, turning once.

Makes one serving

P ER SERVING: 1 G RAIN

Garlic Pita Chips

> 1-ounce pita bread
> ¼ teaspoon garlic powder or garlic salt

Open the pita bread to form 2 rounds. Cut into wedges and sprinkle with the garlic powder or garlic salt. Bake until crisp in a 400° F. oven, about 5 to 8 minutes.

Makes one serving

P ER SERVING: 1 G RAIN

Garlic Soup

Garlic Soup is a Castilian specialty—and a reputed remedy for a hangover. Don't be alarmed by the amount of garlic, a whole head. Cooking greatly reduces its pungency. Note: To make a vegetarian garlic soup, simply omit the ham and use vegetable stock.

> 4 teaspoons olive oil
> 1 head garlic, broken into cloves, peeled, and thinly sliced widthwise

1 ounce lean prosciutto ham or Canadian bacon, cut into matchstick
   slivers (optional)
1 tablespoon Spanish paprika
4 cups vegetable or defatted chicken stock
Salt and freshly ground black pepper
4 1-inch-thick slices of French bread
2 tablespoons chopped flat-leaf parsley

1. Heat the olive oil in a large nonstick saucepan. Add the garlic and cook
over medium heat until lightly browned, about 2 minutes. Stir in the ham
and paprika and cook for 1 minute. Add the stock and bring to a boil.
Simmer the soup until richly flavored, about 5 minutes. Add salt and pepper
to taste.
2. Meanwhile, darkly toast the bread in a toaster or under the broiler. (Dark
toasting gives the bread a smoky flavor, which makes the soup taste richer,
too.)
 3. To serve, place a slice of bread in each of 4 soup bowls. (The soup would
be served in an earthenware bowl in Spain.) Ladle the soup on top, sprinkle
with parsley, and serve.

Makes four 1-cup servings

PER SERVING: 1 GRAIN, 1 EXTRA

Bulgur Salad with Tomato and Mint

Bulgur (cracked wheat) is a great grain for summer. You don't even have to
turn on the stove to cook it: you simply soak it in cold water until tender.
This takes about 8 hours. Start soaking the bulgur before you go to work, so
it will be ready when you come home for dinner. Then the salad can be
assembled in a matter of minutes.
Note: This recipe calls for more salad than you'll need for dinner. The extra
will be used in Bulgur Lettuce Roll-Up with Spicy Yogurt Dipping Sauce
(page 278), which you can prepare for lunch the following day.

2 cups bulgur
2 cucumbers, seeded and diced

2 ripe tomatoes, seeded and diced

1/2 cup finely chopped flat-leaf parsley,
   plus 4 sprigs for garnish

1/3 cup chopped fresh mint (or 1 tablespoon dried)

4 scallions, finely chopped

1 garlic clove, minced

1/4 cup fresh lemon juice

1/2 teaspoon ground cumin

Salt and freshly ground black pepper

4 lettuce leaves, for serving

1. Rinse the bulgur in a strainer and transfer to a large bowl. Add 4 cups cold water. Let soak in the refrigerator until tender and tripled in bulk, 6 to 8 hours.

2. Drain the bulgur in a strainer, pressing with the back of a spoon to extract the excess water. Combine the bulgur, cucumber, tomatoes, parsley, mint, scallions, garlic, lemon juice, and cumin in a mixing bowl and toss to mix. Add salt, pepper, and cumin to taste. Set 1 cup of salad aside for lunch.

3. To serve, place a lettuce leaf on each of 4 salad plates. Mound the bulgur salad in the center and garnish each serving with a sprig of parsley.

Note: To seed a cucumber, cut it in half lengthwise and scrape out the seeds with a melon baller or spoon.

Makes four 1 1/2-cup dinner servings and one 1-cup lunch serving

Per lunch serving: 1 Grain, 1 Vegetable

Per dinner serving: 2 Grains, 1 Vegetable

Bulgur Lettuce Roll-Up
with Spicy Yogurt Dipping Sauce

I like to think of this quick, easy lunch as a Middle Eastern burrito. The filling is leftover bulgur salad.

Roll-Up

3 large lettuce leaves (romaine or Boston)

1 cup Bulgur Salad with Tomato and Mint (page 277)

1 carrot, thinly sliced lengthwise
1 celery stalk, thinly sliced lengthwise
$^1/_2$ red bell pepper, thinly sliced
1 scallion, trimmed
$^1/_2$ tomato, cut into wedges

Yogurt Dipping Sauce

$^1/_2$ cup plain non-fat yogurt
$^1/_2$ garlic clove, minced
$^1/_4$ teaspoon grated lemon zest
$^1/_4$ teaspoon ground cumin
$^1/_4$ teaspoon hot paprika or cayenne
Salt and freshly ground black pepper

1. To make the roll-up, lay the lettuce leaves on a cutting board, one slightly overlapping the other. Spread the bulgur salad in the center. Lay the sliced carrot, celery, pepper, scallion, and tomato on top, running lengthwise. Starting at the side, roll the lettuce into a compact roll.
2. To make the sauce: In a small bowl, whisk together the yogurt, garlic, lemon zest, cumin, and paprika, adding salt and pepper to taste. Use the sauce as a dip for the lettuce roll as you eat it.

Makes one serving

PER SERVING: 1 GRAIN, 2 VEGETABLE, $^1/_2$ DAIRY

Mexican Bean Salad with Pumpkin Seeds

This salad is bursting with south-of-the-border colors and flavors. It's simple, too—and I think you'll find the combination of kidney beans and pumpkin seeds unexpectedly delicious.

4 cups cooked pinto or kidney beans
(if canned, rinse well to remove excess salt)
2 ounces toasted pumpkin seeds
1 yellow bell pepper, diced
1 cucumber, seeded and diced

1/2 red onion, diced

1 to 2 jalapeño chilies, finely chopped
(for a milder salad, seed the chilies)

3 tablespoons chopped fresh cilantro

2 tablespoons red wine vinegar

1 tablespoon lime juice

4 teaspoons olive oil

2 teaspoons brown sugar

Salt and freshly ground black pepper

Drain the beans in a colander, rinse well, and drain again. Combine the beans with the other ingredients in a bowl and toss to mix. Correct the seasoning, adding lime juice or salt to taste.

Makes 6 cups or four 1 1/2-cup servings

Per serving: 3 Proteins, 1 Vegetable, 2 Extras

Gazpacho Salad

Gazpacho is the world's most famous chilled soup. The unique combination of vegetables thickened with diced bread set me thinking about a salad that could be made with these ingredients.

2 tablespoons red wine vinegar

3 tablespoons vegetable or defatted chicken stock

4 teaspoons extra-virgin olive oil

Salt and freshly ground black pepper

1 cucumber, peeled, seeded, and cut into 1/2-inch dice

2 juicy ripe tomatoes, cut into 1/2-inch dice

1 green bell pepper, cut into 1/2-inch dice

2 celery stalks, cut into 1/2-inch pieces

1/2 red onion, finely chopped

1 to 2 garlic cloves, minced

4 slices country-style bread, cut into 1/2-inch cubes

1. In a salad bowl, whisk together the vinegar, stock, and oil. Add salt and pepper to taste.

2. Stir in the cucumber, tomatoes, pepper, celery, onion, garlic, and bread. Let the salad stand for 10 minutes. Correct the seasoning, adding salt or vinegar to taste.

Makes four 1¹/₂- to 2-cup servings

PER SERVING: 1 GRAIN, 1 VEGETABLE, 1 EXTRA

San Antonio Slaw

Jicama is a Mexican root vegetable that tastes like a cross between an apple and a potato. It's very crisp, very refreshing, and a great way to fill up without fat.

> 2 cups shredded green or savoy cabbage
> 1 cup slivered jicama
> ¹/₂ cup slivered mango or peach (about ¹/₂ large peach or mango)
> 1 poblano chili or ¹/₂ green bell pepper, thinly slivered
> 1 carrot, thinly slivered
> ¹/₄ cup chopped fresh cilantro
> 3 tablespoons diced red onion
> 1 to 4 fresh or pickled jalapeño chilies, thinly sliced (the hotter, the better!)
> 1 garlic clove, minced
> 3 tablespoons fresh lime juice, or to taste
> 1 tablespoon honey
> Salt and freshly ground black pepper

Combine all the ingredients in a mixing bowl and toss to mix. Correct the seasoning, adding salt, sugar, or lime juice to taste.

Makes 4 cups or four 1-cup servings

PER SERVING: 1 VEGETABLE OR NEXT-TO-NOTHING

Fusilli Salad with Cherry Tomatoes and Arugula

Arugula (a salad green in the radish family) gives this pasta salad a distinctive peppery bite. Fusilli are coiled or spring-shaped pasta that come in 3-inch lengths.

> 2 cups dried fusilli
> Salt
> 1¹/₂ tablespoons balsamic vinegar
> 1¹/₂ tablespoons vegetable or defatted chicken stock
> 4 teaspoons extra-virgin olive oil
> 1 garlic clove, minced
> Freshly ground black pepper
> 2 cups ripe cherry tomatoes, stemmed and cut in half
> 1 large bunch arugula, washed, dried, and cut crosswise into ¹/₂-inch strips
> 1 tablespoon capers, drained
> ¹/₂ teaspoon hot pepper flakes

1. Cook the fusilli in 4 quarts rapidly boiling water until al dente, about 8 minutes. Drain the pasta in a colander, refresh under cold water, and drain well again.

2. In an attractive salad bowl, whisk together the vinegar, stock, oil, garlic, and salt and pepper to taste. (Whisk until the salt crystals are dissolved.) Add the pasta, tomatoes, arugula, capers, and pepper flakes and toss to mix. Correct the seasoning, adding salt or vinegar to taste; the pasta should be highly seasoned.

Makes 4 cups or four 1-cup servings

PER SERVING: 2 GRAINS, 1 VEGETABLE, 1 EXTRA

Lemon Couscous

Couscous looks like a grain, but actually it's a type of pasta. This North African staple has become a North American favorite—in part thanks to how easy it is to prepare. You can find couscous in the grain section of any supermarket.

1 garlic clove, minced
1 shallot or $1/2$ small onion, minced
1 teaspoon grated lemon zest
2 tablespoons chopped parsley
$2^1/2$ cups vegetable or defatted chicken stock
2 cups dry couscous
Salt and freshly ground pepper

1. In a large frying pan, combine the garlic, onion, lemon zest, parsley, and stock and gently simmer for 5 minutes.
2. Remove the pan from the heat and stir in the couscous and salt and pepper to taste. Cover the pan and let stand for 10 minutes, or until the couscous is soft. Fluff the couscous with a fork before serving, adding salt and pepper to taste.

Makes four 1-cup servings

PER SERVING: 2 GRAINS

Poppy Seed Noodles

4 cups cooked noodles
$1/4$ cup non-fat sour cream
2 teaspoons poppy seeds

Toss the noodles with the sour cream and poppy seeds.

Makes four 1-cup servings

PER SERVING: 2 GRAINS

Roast Beef Sandwich

    1 slice of sourdough bread
    $^1/_2$ teaspoon grainy mustard
    $^1/_2$ teaspoon prepared horseradish
    3 lettuce leaves
    1 ounce roast beef
    3 tomato slices
    1 cup radish or alfalfa sprouts

Generously spread a slice of sourdough bread with grainy mustard and pre-pared horseradish. Place the lettuce leaves and roast beef on top. Top the sandwich with the tomato slices and sprouts.

Makes one serving

PER SERVING: 1 GRAIN, 1 PROTEIN

Greek Salad Sandwich

    1-ounce pita bread
    Romaine lettuce
    Tomato slices
    Sliced red onion
    Chopped scallions
    Fresh dill sprigs
    1 tablespoon lemon juice
    1 ounce feta cheese

Stuff a pita bread with romaine lettuce leaves, tomato slices, sliced red onion, chopped scallions, and fresh dill sprigs. Sprinkle with lemon juice and crumbled feta cheese.

Makes one serving

PER SERVING: 1 GRAIN, 1 VEGETABLE, 1 DAIRY, 1 EXTRA

Veggie Melt

1 slice of pumpernickel bread
Spicy mustard
3 tomato slices
3 jicama slices
1 ounce low-fat American or cheddar cheese
Freshly ground black pepper

Spread a slice of pumpernickel with spicy mustard. Top with the tomato and jicama slices. Place cheese on top and sprinkle with freshly ground black pepper. Cook under a broiler or in a toaster oven to melt the cheese.

Makes one serving

Per serving: 1 Grain, 1 Dairy, 1 Vegetable (or count vegetables as Next-to-Nothing)

Portobello-Goat Cheese Sandwich

1 portobello mushroom cap
1 garlic clove, slivered
Salt and freshly ground pepper
2-ounce multigrain roll
1 ounce softened goat cheese
1/2 bunch watercress
3 slices of tomato

Stud a portobello mushroom cap with slivers of garlic and season with salt and pepper. Grill or broil the mushroom until nicely browned and tender, about 4 minutes per side. Cut the multigrain roll in half, spread with the softened goat cheese, and fill with the mushroom, watercress, and tomato slices.

Makes one serving

Per serving: 2 Grains, 1 Dairy, 1 Extra

Chicken Paprikas

Here's a low-fat remake of a Hungarian classic. For the best results, use imported Hungarian paprika, which is available at gourmet shops and many supermarkets.

1 pound skinless, boneless chicken breasts,
   thinly sliced across the grain
Salt and freshly ground black pepper
1 tablespoon sweet paprika (or to taste)
2 teaspoons olive oil
1 onion, finely chopped
2 garlic cloves, finely chopped
1 red bell pepper, finely chopped
1 tomato, finely chopped
1 tablespoon flour
1 cup defatted chicken stock
3/4 cup non-fat sour cream
2 tablespoons chopped flat-leaf parsley, for garnish (optional)

1. Place the chicken in a bowl and season with salt, pepper, and half the paprika. Toss to mix. Let stand for 5 minutes.

2. Meanwhile, heat the oil in a large nonstick sauté pan or skillet. Add the onion, garlic, and pepper and cook over medium heat until the vegetables are soft and just beginning to brown, about 5 minutes, stirring often. Add the tomato after 3 minutes. Stir in the flour and remaining paprika and cook for 1 minute.

3. Stir in the chicken and cook for 1 minute. Stir in the stock and most of the sour cream, reserving 2 tablespoons for garnish. Gently simmer until the chicken is cooked and the sauce is nicely thickened, 8 to 10 minutes. Add salt, pepper, and paprika as needed to taste.

4. Transfer the paprikas to plates or a platter. Garnish with dollops of sour cream sprinkled with parsley, if desired.

Makes four servings

PER SERVING: 4 PROTEINS, 1 VEGETABLE, 2 EXTRAS

Spaghetti Primavera with Grilled Vegetables

One of the best ways to create big, mouth-watering flavors with a minimum of fat is to use cooking methods that add flavor, like grilling. These grilled vegetables give this pasta so much flavor, you won't miss the heavy cream in the original. The sauce is made by simmering stock and non-fat sour cream.

Grilled Vegetables

  1 zucchini, cut on the diagonal into ¼-inch slices
  1 yellow squash, cut on the diagonal into ¼-inch slices
  1 onion, cut into ¼-inch slices
  Olive oil spray (or a paper towel dipped in 1 teaspoon olive oil)
  Salt and freshly ground black pepper

  4 ounces spaghetti
  Salt

Sauce

  4 teaspoons extra-virgin olive oil
  2 shallots, finely chopped
  2 garlic cloves, finely chopped
  1 tomato, seeded and finely chopped
  1 cup vegetable or defatted chicken stock
  1 cup non-fat sour cream
  8 fresh basil leaves, thinly slivered, plus 4 whole leaves for garnish
  Freshly ground black pepper and a pinch of cayenne

  3 ounces freshly grated Parmesan cheese

1. Preheat the barbecue grill or broiler. Spray the zucchini, squash, and onion slices with oil (or wipe them with an oiled paper towel). Season with salt and pepper to taste. Grill the zucchini, squash, and onion slices until nicely browned on both sides, 3 to 4 minutes per side. Transfer to a platter.
2. Cook the pasta in 3 quarts lightly salted, boiling water until al dente, 8 minutes.
3. Meanwhile, heat the olive oil in a nonstick skillet. Cook the shallots and garlic until fragrant but not brown, about 2 minutes. Add the tomato and cook for 1 minute. Thinly slice the grilled vegetables, add them to the pan, and cook for 1 minute.

4. Add the chicken stock and sour cream. Briskly boil for 5 to 8 minutes, or until well reduced, thickened, and richly flavored. Stir in the basil and pasta and cook until thoroughly heated, 2 minutes, turning with tongs. Correct the seasoning, adding salt and peppers to taste.

5. Spoon the pasta into bowls and sprinkle with the cheese.

Makes four servings

Per serving: 1 Grain, 1 Dairy, 1 Vegetable, 1 Extra

Paella Valenciana

Paella is a colorful Spanish rice stew that makes a great dish for entertaining. You'll need to know about one special ingredient: Valencia-style rice, a short, starchy grain similar to Italian arborio. Look for it in the rice section of your supermarket (especially if your supermarket caters to a large Hispanic clientele) or use arborio rice.

  1 tablespoon extra-virgin olive oil
  1 onion, finely chopped
  2 garlic cloves, minced
  $1/2$ red bell pepper, cut into $1/4$-inch strips
  $1/2$ yellow bell pepper, cut into $1/4$-inch strips
  1 ripe tomato, seeded and cut into $1/4$-inch dice
  6 ounces skinless, boneless chicken breasts, cut into 1-inch pieces
  2 cups Valencia-style rice
  $1/2$ cup dry white wine
  5 cups vegetable or defatted chicken stock, or as needed
  $1/2$ teaspoon saffron threads, soaked in 1 tablespoon hot water
      for 15 minutes
  12 littleneck clams, scrubbed
  12 mussels, scrubbed
  12 ounces shrimp, peeled and deveined
  $1/2$ cup cooked green peas
  2 tablespoons flat-leaf parsley

1. Heat the olive oil in a large, heavy, handsome skillet. (I use a cast-iron skillet that looks attractive when I bring it to the table.) Sauté the onion, garlic, and peppers over medium heat until golden brown, 6 minutes, stirring often. Increase the heat to high, add the tomato, and cook for 1 minute. Add the chicken pieces and lightly brown. Transfer the chicken to a plate with tongs and set aside.

2. Add the rice and sauté until the grains are shiny, 1 minute. Add the wine and bring to a boil. Add the stock and saffron and bring to a boil. Reduce the heat and simmer the rice, uncovered, for 10 minutes. Stir in the chicken, clams, and mussels, and simmer for 5 minutes. Add the shrimp and simmer for 5 to 8 minutes, or until the chicken and shrimp are cooked through, the clam and mussel shells have opened, and the rice is tender. Stir in the peas. The paella should be quite moist; if the rice starts to dry out, add a little more stock or water.

3. Just before serving, correct the seasoning, adding salt and pepper to taste. Sprinkle with the parsley and serve at once.

Makes four servings

PER SERVING: 4 PROTEINS, 2 GRAINS, 1 VEGETABLE, 1 EXTRA

Three-Bean Chili

Here's a vegetarian chili that's as colorful as it is tasty. Don't be alarmed by the large number of ingredients. The recipe can be assembled in 20 minutes—even less if you chop the vegetables in a food processor. If you use canned beans, rinse well to remove excess salt.

1 tablespoon olive oil
1 onion, finely chopped
2 garlic cloves, finely chopped
1/2 green bell pepper, finely chopped
1 jalapeño chili, seeded and finely chopped
1 celery stalk, very finely chopped
1 to 2 tablespoons chili powder (or to taste)
1/2 teaspoon ground cumin
1/2 teaspoon dried oregano

2 cups cooked red kidney beans

2 cups cooked white beans

2 cups cooked garbanzo beans

8 ounces firm tofu, crumbled

1 14-ounce can peeled tomatoes, pureed with their juices

1 cup vegetable stock

$1/2$ teaspoon Tabasco sauce (or to taste)

Salt and freshly ground black pepper

1 tablespoon coarse yellow cornmeal

2 chopped scallions, for garnish

1. Heat the olive oil in a large heavy pot. Add the chopped vegetables and brown over medium heat, about 6 minutes. Add the spices and cook for 1 minute.

2. Stir in the beans, tofu, tomatoes with juices, stock, Tabasco sauce, and salt and pepper to taste. Simmer the chili, uncovered, until thick and flavorful, about 10 minutes. Stir in the cornmeal in a thin stream to thicken the chili and cook for 1 minute. Correct the seasoning, adding salt and pepper to taste.

3. To serve, ladle the chili into bowls and garnish with a sprinkling of chopped scallions.

Makes 8 cups or four 2-cup servings

Per serving: 4 Proteins, 1 Vegetable, 1 Extra

Teriyaki Salmon with Spicy Slaw

This colorful salmon dish is a favorite supper at our house. Rice vinegar (available at most supermarkets) has a milder flavor than regular vinegar. If unavailable, use 3 tablespoons distilled white vinegar and 1 tablespoon water. Black sesame seeds and sesame oil are sold at health food stores and Asian markets.

Spicy Slaw

1 garlic clove, minced

1 tablespoon minced fresh ginger

1 scallion, finely chopped

$^1/_4$ cup rice vinegar

1 tablespoon sugar

$^1/_2$ teaspoon of your favorite hot sauce (optional)

3 cups thinly sliced napa (Chinese cabbage) or savoy cabbage

$^1/_2$ red bell pepper, thinly sliced

1 carrot, shredded

1 tablespoon black sesame seeds or poppy seeds

Salt and freshly ground black pepper

Teriyaki Salmon

$^1/_2$ teaspoon sesame oil or olive oil (on a paper towel)

$1^1/_2$ pounds skinless, boneless salmon fillets, cut into
four 6-ounce portions

$^1/_4$ cup teriyaki sauce

1. Prepare the slaw: In a mixing bowl, combine the garlic, ginger, scallion, vinegar, sugar, and hot sauce. Whisk until the sugar is dissolved. Add the cabbage, pepper, carrot, and sesame seeds and toss to mix. Add salt and pepper to taste.

2. Preheat the broiler. Set the top rack about 5 inches below the heat. Preheat a baking dish you've lightly oiled with sesame oil. Season the fish with salt and pepper and place in the preheated baking dish. Lightly brush the top with teriyaki sauce. Broil the salmon until almost cooked, 6 to 8 minutes. Brush the remaining teriyaki sauce on the salmon and continue broiling until the fish is cooked through and the top is shiny and brown, 2 to 4 minutes more.

3. To serve, mound the slaw on plates. Place a piece of fish in the center of each.

Makes four servings

PER SERVING: 4 PROTEINS, 1 VEGETABLE, 1 EXTRA

Bouillabaisse with Garlic Toasts

Bouillabaisse is the world's most famous fish stew, a brimming bowl chock full of seafood and vegetables, perfumed with anise, orange, and saffron. Once you've assembled the ingredients, this recipe can be prepared in less than 30 minutes. Note: Feel free to vary the seafood, using what looks freshest and best at the market.

Bouillabaisse

$^1/_2$ cup dry white wine

1 onion, finely chopped

1 leek, washed, trimmed, and finely chopped

3 garlic cloves, minced

1 teaspoon dried oregano

1 teaspoon fennel seeds

$^1/_4$ cup fresh orange juice, plus 2 strips of orange zest

1 14-ounce can peeled tomatoes, pureed with juices

5 cups bottled clam juice or defatted chicken broth

1 cup water

$^1/_2$ teaspoon saffron, soaked in 1 tablespoon hot water for
   15 minutes

2 medium potatoes, peeled and cut into 1-inch pieces

18 mussels

18 littleneck clams (or $^1/_2$ pound sliced squid)

12 ounces shrimp, peeled and deveined

12 ounces skinless, boneless white fish fillets, such as cod or snapper,
   cut into 2-inch pieces

Salt and freshly ground black pepper

Garlic Toasts

6 slices of French bread, cut sharply on the diagonal

1 garlic clove, cut in half

2 tablespoons chopped fresh parsley

1. Bring the wine to a boil in a large pot. Add the onion, leek, garlic, oregano, and fennel seeds and briskly simmer until the vegetables are soft, about 3 minutes. Stir in the orange juice and zest and bring to a boil. Add the tomatoes and return to a boil. Transfer this mixture to a food processor

or blender and puree. Return it to the pot. Or leave the mixture as is—chunky bouillabaisse is delicious.

2. Add the clam juice, water, saffron, and potatoes. Briskly simmer for 5 minutes, or until the potatoes are half cooked. Stir in the mussels and clams and simmer for 3 minutes. Stir in the shrimp and fish and simmer for 5 minutes, or until the potatoes are tender and all the seafood is cooked. Add salt and pepper to taste.

3. Meanwhile, make the toasts: Darkly toast the bread slices in a toaster, toaster oven, or under the broiler. Transfer to a cake rack to cool. Rub each toast with the cut garlic.

4. To serve the bouillabaisse, ladle the broth and seafood into bowls. Sprinkle with parsley. Place a toast on top of each, half in the bowl, half over the edge, and serve at once.

Makes six servings

PER SERVING: 3 PROTEINS, 1 GRAIN, 2 VEGETABLES

Moroccan Lamb Kebabs

Cumin, coriander, and saffron give these kebabs a Moroccan accent. Serve with Lemon Couscous (page 283).

> 1 pound lean leg of lamb, cut into 1-inch chunks
> $^1/_2$ teaspoon ground cumin
> $^1/_2$ teaspoon ground coriander
> $^1/_4$ teaspoon saffron threads (crumbled between your fingers)
> Salt and freshly ground black pepper
> 3 tablespoons fresh lemon juice
> 8 mushrooms
> 8 pearl onions
> 8 cherry tomatoes
> 1 green bell pepper, cut into 1-inch pieces

Garnish
> 2 tablespoons chopped parsley
> 1 lemon, cut into 4 wedges

1. Combine the lamb, cumin, coriander, saffron, and salt and pepper in a bowl and toss to mix. Stir in the lemon juice. Let marinate 30 minutes.

2. Preheat the grill or broiler to high. Thread the lamb onto skewers, alternating with the mushrooms, onions, cherry tomatoes, and bell pepper pieces. Grill the kebabs until cooked, about 8 minutes in all. Transfer to a platter and sprinkle with the parsley, serving the lemon wedges on the side. Squeeze lemon juice on the kebabs before eating.

Makes four servings

Per serving: 4 Proteins, 1 Vegetable

Spicy Ginger Turkey Stir-Fry

This gingery stir-fry is so chock full of flavor you won't miss the fat. The recipe uses a technique I call "broth-frying": The ingredients are cooked in sizzling chicken stock instead of oil. You can easily create different versions of this recipe by using tofu, chicken, or meat instead of turkey and substituting other combinations of vegetables. As with all stir-fries, have all the ingredients chopped, measured out, and ready to go before you start cooking.

> 12 ounces lean turkey breast

Sauce
> 1/4 cup vegetable or defatted chicken stock, plus 1/4 cup for stir-frying
> 2 tablespoons rice wine or sherry
> 1 1/2 tablespoons soy sauce
> 1 1/2 tablespoons oyster sauce (see Note)
> 2 teaspoons sugar
> 1 tablespoon cornstarch

> 2 tablespoons minced fresh ginger
> 3 garlic cloves, minced
> 3 scallions, white part minced, green part cut into 1-inch pieces for garnish
> 2 cups stir-fry vegetables (use a mix of carrots, cabbage, celery, and broccoli; the selection and precise amounts of each are flexible)

1. Cut the turkey across the grain into strips 2 inches long, 1 inch wide, and 1/8 inch thick.

2. Combine the ingredients for the sauce in a small bowl and stir until the cornstarch is dissolved.

3. Just before serving, bring the remaining 1/4 cup stock to a boil in a non-stick wok or skillet over high heat. Add the ginger, garlic, and scallion whites and stir-fry until fragrant, about 30 seconds. Add the turkey and vegetables and stir-fry until the turkey is almost cooked and the vegetables are almost tender, about 3 minutes. Stir the sauce again to redissolve the cornstarch and add it to the wok. Continue stir-frying until the turkey is cooked and nicely coated with sauce, 1 to 2 minutes. Sprinkle with the scallion greens and serve at once.

Note: Oyster sauce is a thick, sweet, salty sauce flavored with oysters. If unavailable, substitute 1 tablespoon soy sauce and 1 teaspoon brown sugar.

Makes four 1 1/4- to 1 1/2-cup servings

PER SERVING: 3 PROTEINS, 1 VEGETABLE

Shabu-Shabu (Japanese Fondue) with Lemon-Ginger Dipping Sauce

Shabu-Shabu is the Japanese version of fondue or Mongolian hot pot. The name is said to echo the sound that the ingredients make as they swish through the broth. The traditional recipe calls for the broth to be flavored with kombu (dried kelp). I've opted for more readily available flavorings, such as ginger and garlic. One of the best things about Shabu-Shabu is that once the ingredients are cooked, you get to enjoy the broth as a soup.

Broth

> 6 cups vegetable or defatted chicken stock
> 4 dried black mushrooms (shiitakes)
> 2 1/4-inch-thick fresh ginger slices, flattened with the side of a knife or cleaver
> 2 garlic cloves, thinly sliced
> 2 scallions, thinly sliced

Ingredients for dipping

6 to 8 lettuce leaves, washed, for lining the serving platter

6 ounces firm tofu, thinly sliced

6 ounces skinless, boneless chicken breast, thinly sliced

6 ounces shrimp, peeled and deveined

2 cups fresh spinach, washed and stemmed

2 cups sliced napa cabbage leaves, cut into 2-inch pieces
(or substitute green or savoy cabbage)

2 cups broccoli florets

4 carrots, very thinly sliced on the diagonal

1 large sweet potato, peeled and thinly sliced

Lemon-Ginger Dipping Sauce

$1/2$ cup fresh lemon juice

$1/2$ teaspoon grated lemon zest

$1/3$ cup tamari (or substitute soy sauce)

$1/4$ cup water

2 tablespoons sugar

2 garlic cloves, minced

2 teaspoons grated fresh ginger

2 scallions, finely chopped

$1/4$ teaspoon hot pepper flakes

Salt and freshly ground pepper

1. Combine the stock, black mushrooms, ginger, garlic, and scallions in a fondue pot and simmer for 10 minutes. Remove the mushrooms with a slotted spoon; discard the stems and set mushroom caps aside.

2. Line a large platter with lettuce leaves. Arrange the tofu, chicken, shrimp, spinach, napa, broccoli, carrots, sweet potato, and mushroom caps in neat piles on top. The Shabu-Shabu can be prepared ahead to this stage and refrigerated.

3. Combine the dipping sauce ingredients in a bowl and stir to mix.

4. Provide each guest with a plate, a small bowl of dipping sauce, and a set of chopsticks or a fondue fork. Have the broth simmering in a fondue pot (or saucepan on a tabletop burner) in the center of the table. Have each guest dip the chicken, shrimp, and vegetables in the simmering broth and cook

them to taste, 1 to 3 minutes, depending on the item. Important note: Since the vegetables—including the decorative lettuce leaves—have come into contact with raw poultry and shrimp, they should not be eaten unless they're first cooked in the broth.

5. After the dipping ingredients are all cooked, take the broth to the kitchen. Season with salt and pepper, strain into mugs, and serve as soup.

Makes four servings

PER SERVING: 3 PROTEINS, 2 VEGETABLES, 1 EXTRA

Fish en Papillote

Few dishes offer more drama with less preparation time than Fish en Papillote. The fish is baked with vegetables and fresh herbs in an aluminum foil pouch, which puffs theatrically for serving. The foil seals in all the flavor, creating a great-tasting meal with no added fat. I've called for snapper here, but you could use any fresh fish.

> 2 potatoes (about 1 pound), peeled and thinly sliced
> Salt and freshly ground black pepper
> 4 6-ounce pieces of snapper or other fish
> 1 tomato, cut into $1/4$-inch dice
> 1 zucchini, cut into $1/4$-inch dice
> 1 yellow squash, cut into $1/4$-inch dice
> 1 red bell pepper, cut into $1/4$-inch dice
> 4 fresh basil leaves (or 1 teaspoon dried)
> 4 bay leaves
> $1/2$ cup dry white vermouth or wine

1. Preheat the oven to 400° F. Arrange 4 large (12 by 20 inches) rectangles of heavy-duty foil on a work surface, shiny side down. In the center of each, spread out a quarter of the sliced potatoes. Season with salt and pepper. Place a piece of fish on top and season with salt and pepper. Arrange a quarter of the diced tomatoes, zucchini, squash, and pepper, and a basil and a bay leaf on top. Sprinkle with a little more salt and pepper.

2. For each serving, bring together the short edges of the foil rectangle high

over the fish. Pour 2 tablespoons of wine over each piece of fish. Crimp the top edges of the foil to form an airtight seal.

3. Place the papillotes on baking sheets and bake until the foil is puffed and the fish inside is cooked, about 20 minutes. Serve the papillotes on plates. Help each guest open the packet and slide the fish, vegetables, and juices onto the plate. Take care not to burn yourselves on the escaping steam.

Makes four servings

PER SERVING: 3 PROTEINS, 1 VEGETABLE

Melon Salad with Yogurt and Mint

This refreshing fruit salad offers the unexpected flavor combination of ginger and fresh mint.

> 1 cup plain non-fat yogurt
> $1/2$ teaspoon ground ginger
> $1/2$ teaspoon ground cinnamon
> 2 tablespoons brown sugar
> 2 tablespoons fresh lime juice
> 4 cups cubed cantaloupe or honeydew melon
> 3 tablespoons slivered fresh mint leaves,
>   plus 4 whole sprigs for garnish

1. In a mixing bowl, whisk together the yogurt, ginger, cinnamon, brown sugar, and lime juice. Stir in the melon and mint.

2. Transfer the salad to wineglasses or bowls and garnish each with a sprig of fresh mint.

Makes four 1-cup servings

PER SERVING: 1 FRUIT, 1 EXTRA

Orange Custard

This egg-rich dessert might seem like an unlikely candidate for a low-fat makeover. But by using fat-free dairy products and egg whites instead of whole eggs, we can slash the fat to almost nothing. The orange flavor comes through loud and clear thanks to the addition of grated orange zest, orange liqueur, and a perfumed flavoring called orange flower water. The latter is available in Middle Eastern markets.

1 14-ounce can fat-free sweetened condensed milk
10 ounces (1^1/8 cups) skim milk
12 egg whites (or 1^1/4 cups egg substitute)
1 tablespoon Grand Marnier or other orange liqueur
1 tablespoon orange flower water (or 1 teaspoon orange extract)
1 teaspoon vanilla extract
1 teaspoon freshly grated orange zest
^{1}/2 teaspoon ground cinnamon
Pinch of salt

6 6-ounce ramekins or custard cups

1. Preheat the oven to 350° F. Bring 1 quart water to a boil.
2. In a mixing bowl, whisk together the condensed milk, skim milk, egg whites, orange liqueur, orange flower water, vanilla, orange zest, cinnamon, and salt. Ladle this mixture into the ramekins. Set the ramekins in a roasting pan, pour ^{1}/2 inch boiling water around them, and place in the oven. Bake 30 to 40 minutes, or until the custards are set. Transfer the custards to a rack to cool, then refrigerate for at least 4 hours, preferably overnight. Serve cold.

Makes six servings

Per serving: 1 Dairy, 1 Protein, 2 Extras

Coconut Fruit Salad

Toasted coconut adds a tropical touch to this colorful fruit salad. Feel free to replace any of the fruits mentioned below with other fruits.

> 1 starfruit, thinly sliced
> 1 banana, peeled and diced
> 2 kiwifruits, peeled and diced
> 1 cup fresh blueberries
> 1 orange, peeled and cut or broken into segments
> 2 tablespoons coconut rum (such as Malibu) or orange liqueur
> 2 tablespoons lightly toasted coconut

1. Set 4 starfruit slices aside for garnish. (Make a slit in each so it will slip over the edge of a glass.) Combine the remaining fruit and rum in a mixing bowl and gently toss to mix.
2. Spoon the fruit into wine or martini glasses. Sprinkle each salad with a little toasted coconut. Slide a starfruit slice over the edge of each glass and serve at once.
Note: It's easy to toast your own coconut. Just buy sweetened grated coconut in the supermarket and toast it in a thin layer on a baking sheet in a 400° F. oven until golden brown, about 5 minutes.

Makes four 1-cup servings

PER SERVING: 1 FRUIT, 1 EXTRA

Blueberry Soup

Here's a colorful soup that's as refreshing as it is unexpected. My favorite berry is the tiny Maine blueberry, which is in season in August. (In a pinch you can use frozen.)

> 3 cups fresh blueberries
> 1 cup cranberry juice cocktail
> 1 1/2 cups water
> 3 ounces (6 tablespoons) white wine
> 1 tablespoon sugar (or to taste)

2 teaspoons minced fresh ginger

1 cinnamon stick

2 teaspoons cornstarch

3 ounces (6 tablespoons) port wine

8 fresh mint leaves, cut into thin slivers

1. Pick through the berries, removing any stems. Wash well. Place the berries, cranberry juice, water, white wine, sugar, ginger, and cinnamon stick in a pot and bring to a boil. Simmer the blueberries for 5 minutes.

2. Dissolve the cornstarch in the port wine and whisk the mixture into the berries. Simmer for 3 minutes. Discard the cinnamon stick and puree the soup in a blender. Or leave the soup chunky if you prefer. Transfer to a bowl and allow to cool to room temperature, then refrigerate until cold. If too thick, thin with a little water.

3. To serve, ladle the soup into wine goblets or brandy snifters. Sprinkle the mint on top and serve.

Makes four servings

PER SERVING: 1 FRUIT, 1 EXTRA

Strawberry Napoleons

Here's a stunning dessert for entertaining that has only a fraction of the fat found in the traditional recipe. The secret is to use an unexpected ingredient—a baked wonton wrapper—to make the pastry. Wonton wrappers are available in the produce section of most supermarkets. Or use egg roll wrappers, cutting them into 3-inch squares. Don't be intimidated by the length of the recipe. It's really just a series of simple steps.

Pastry

Oil cooking spray

12 wonton wrappers (each about 3 inches square)

4 teaspoons granulated sugar

1/2 teaspoon cinnamon

Pastry Cream

    1 cup skim milk

    3 tablespoons granulated sugar

    1¹/₂ tablespoons cornstarch

    1 egg

    1 teaspoon orange liqueur

    ¹/₂ teaspoon vanilla extract

    ¹/₂ teaspoon grated lemon zest

    2 pints strawberries

    1 tablespoon confectioners' sugar

1. Prepare the pastry: preheat the oven to 400° F. Lightly spray a nonstick baking sheet with oil. Arrange the wonton wrappers on top and lightly spray with oil. Mix the 4 teaspoons of sugar and cinnamon in a small bowl and lightly sprinkle this mixture over the wonton wrappers. Bake the wrappers until golden brown and crisp, about 5 minutes. Transfer the wrappers to a cake rack to cool. The pastry tastes best served within 2 hours of being baked. If you wish to prepare it further ahead of time—or even the day before—store it in an airtight tin to keep it from getting soggy.

2. Prepare the pastry cream: heat the milk in a saucepan and gradually bring to a boil, stirring often to prevent scorching. Meanwhile, in a mixing bowl, whisk together the 3 tablespoons sugar and the cornstarch. Add the egg and whisk to mix. Whisk the scalded milk into the egg mix in a thin stream. Return the mix to the pan and bring to a boil, whisking steadily.

3. Reduce the heat and cook until thickened, about 2 minutes. The mixture should bubble. Transfer the pastry cream to a bowl and whisk in the orange liqueur, vanilla extract, and lemon zest. Press a piece of plastic wrap on top of the cream to prevent a skin from forming, making a slit in the top to allow the steam to escape. Let cool to room temperature, then refrigerate until cold. The cream can be made up to 24 hours ahead.

4. Not more than 1 hour before serving, wash, stem, and thinly slice half the strawberries. Leave the remaining berries whole for decoration.

5. Shortly before serving, excuse yourself from the table and assemble the napoleons in the kitchen. (Better yet, invite everyone into the kitchen to watch!) Arrange 4 baked wonton wrappers on a work surface. Gently spread a couple of tablespoons of pastry cream on each wrapper and arrange the

strawberry slices on top. (You should use up half the pastry cream and sliced berries.) Place a second wonton wrapper on top and top with the remaining pastry cream and berries. Place a third wonton wrapper on top. Sift a little confectioners' sugar over each napoleon. Using a spatula, transfer the napoleons to plates. Garnish with the whole berries and serve.

Makes four servings

PER SERVING: 1 GRAIN, 1 FRUIT, 2 EXTRAS

Peaches in Sparkling Wine

>1 ripe peach
>6 ounces sparkling wine

Dice 1 ripe peach into a wineglass. Fill the glass with sparkling wine.

Makes one serving

PER SERVING: 1 FRUIT, 1 EXTRA

Indian Milk Shake

Lassi is the Indian version of a milk shake, a refreshing, nourishing beverage made with yogurt, ice, and rose water, a perfumed flavoring popular in Indian and Middle Eastern cooking. Look for it at gourmet shops, Middle Eastern and Indian markets, and at your local pharmacy.

>1 cup plain non-fat yogurt
>2 teaspoons honey (or to taste)
>$1/2$ teaspoon rose water (or to taste)
>4 ice cubes
>$1/8$ teaspoon ground cardamom

1. Combine the yogurt, honey, rose water, and ice in a blender and blend until smooth. Correct the seasoning, adding honey or rose water to taste.

2. Pour the lassi into a tall glass. Sprinkle the cardamom on top and serve at once.

Makes one serving

Per serving: 1 Dairy, 1 Extra

Fruit Juice Spritzer

3 ounces fruit juice
6 ounces club soda

Combine the fruit juice with the club soda.

Makes one serving

Per serving: ½ Fruit

Lemon-Mint Spritzer

1 tablespoon lemon juice
Lemon slice
Club soda
Fresh mint

Add lemon juice and a lemon slice to a glass of club soda. Add a bruised sprig of fresh mint.

Makes one serving

Per serving: Next-to-Nothing

Peach Yogurt Smoothie

1 peach
1 cup plain non-fat yogurt
2 teaspoons honey
4 ice cubes

Puree the peach, yogurt, honey, and ice cubes in a blender. Serve immediately.

Makes one serving

PER SERVING: 1 FRUIT, 1 DAIRY, 1 EXTRA

Vietnamese Iced Coffee

> 1 cup ice
> 1 tablespoon non-fat sweetened condensed milk
> 1 cup hot coffee

Fill a tall glass with ice. Add the condensed milk. Place a spoon in the glass. Slowly add the hot coffee, pouring it on the spoon to absorb the heat.

Makes one serving

PER SERVING: 1 EXTRA

Café de Olla

Café de Olla is spice-flavored Mexican coffee.

> 1 cup hot coffee
> Pinch of cinnamon
> Pinch of cloves
> 2 teaspoons brown sugar
> $1/2$ teaspoon vanilla extract

To a cup of your favorite coffee, add the cinnamon, cloves, brown sugar, and vanilla.

Makes one serving

PER SERVING: 1 EXTRA

Café Latte

$1/4$ cup espresso or strong coffee
1 cup hot skim milk

Combine the espresso with the hot milk.

Makes one serving

Per serving: 1 Dairy

Mexican Egg Scramble

I like to think of this recipe as a low-fat huevos rancheros. Serve with your favorite fat-free salsa. If you like spicy food, leave the chili seeds in.

4 flour tortillas
4 teaspoons olive oil
1 onion, finely chopped
2 garlic cloves, finely chopped
1 to 2 jalapeño chilies, seeded and finely chopped
1 tomato, seeded and finely chopped
$1/4$ cup chopped fresh cilantro
12 egg whites, lightly beaten (or 1 cup egg substitute)
Salt and freshly ground black pepper
$2/3$ cup of your favorite fat-free salsa

1. Cut each tortilla into 8 wedges. Place on a baking sheet and cook in a 400° F. oven until golden brown, about 5 minutes. Transfer to a rack and let cool.
2. Heat the oil in a nonstick frying pan. Add the onion, garlic, and chilies and cook until the onion is soft but not brown, about 4 minutes. Add the tomato and half the cilantro and cook for 2 minutes. Add the eggs and salt and pepper to taste and cook until scrambled, about 3 minutes. Correct the seasoning, adding salt and pepper to taste.
3. Serve the scramble on plates with the tortilla chips and salsa.

Makes four servings

PER SERVING: 1 PROTEIN, 1 GRAIN, 1 VEGETABLE, 1 EXTRA

Cinnamon-Orange Popovers

Cinnamon, orange zest, and almond extract add so much flavor to these popovers that you won't miss the egg yolks and butter found in traditional recipes. The secret to achieving a dramatic puff is to bake the popovers in deep nonstick molds.

> 1 cup all-purpose unbleached white flour
> $1/2$ teaspoon ground cinnamon
> $1/2$ teaspoon freshly grated orange zest
> $1/2$ teaspoon almond extract
> $1/2$ teaspoon salt
> 1 cup skim milk, at room temperature
> 4 egg whites
> 2 teaspoons canola oil (or substitute another type of oil or melted butter)

> Deep popover molds lightly sprayed or wiped with oil

1. Preheat the oven to 450° F.
2. Combine the ingredients for the popovers in a blender and blend until smooth. Pour the batter into the molds, filling each mold a third full.
3. Bake the popovers for 15 minutes without opening the oven door. Lower the heat to 350° F. and continue baking for 30 minutes, or until the popovers are puffed and well browned. Unmold and serve at once.
Note: If you don't own popover molds, use muffin tins, filling each about halfway. Alternatively, you can bake the batter in a baking dish in the style of Yorkshire pudding.

Makes 6 large popovers, one per serving

PER SERVING: 1 GRAIN, 1 EXTRA

Cream of Wheat Cereal

1 1/2 cups skim milk
1/4 cup cream of wheat
Pinch salt
2 teaspoons blueberry syrup

1. Slowly heat the milk until it reaches a simmer.
2. Stir in cream of wheat and salt. Simmer for about 3 minutes, stirring until the cereal thickens.
3. Serve with blueberry syrup.

Makes one serving

PER SERVING: 1 1/2 DAIRY (OR COUNT AS 1 DAIRY AND 1 PROTEIN), 2 GRAINS, 1 EXTRA

Granola Parfait

This takes just seconds to make, but it really looks terrific. Remember, we eat with our eyes as well as our palates.

1/4 cup non-fat granola
1 cup lemon yogurt
1/2 cup blueberries or raspberries

In a parfait glass or wineglass, layer the granola, yogurt, and berries.

Makes one serving

PER SERVING: 1 DAIRY, 1 GRAIN, 1/2 FRUIT, 2 EXTRAS

INDEX

▼   ▼   ▼   ▼

ABOUT MIRIAM NELSON AND SARAH WERNICK

Authors of *Strong Women Stay Slim* and the national bestseller *Strong Women Stay Young*

Miriam Nelson, Ph.D., is Associate Chief of the Human Physiology Laboratory at the Jean Mayer USDA Human Nutrition Research Center on Aging at Tufts University and Assistant Professor at the School of Nutrition Science and Policy. She is a Fellow of the American College of Sports Medicine and holds their certification as a health/fitness director. Her original research papers have been published in distinguished peer-reviewed journals, including the *Journal of the American Medical Association* and the *New England Journal of Medicine*. She is a former Brookdale National Fellow and is currently a Bunting Fellow at Radcliffe College. She lives in Concord, Massachusetts, with her husband and three children.

Sarah Wernick, Ph.D., is an award-winning freelance writer based in Brookline, Massachusetts. Her articles have appeared in *Woman's Day, Working Mother, Smithsonian,* The *New York Times,* and other publications. She is married and has two children.

The *Strong Women* World Wide Web site is
http://www.strongwomen.com

ABOUT STEVEN RAICHLEN

Steven Raichlen is the author of thirteen cookbooks, winner of a Julia Child/IACP Award, and two-time winner of the James Beard Award for his *High-Flavor, Low-Fat* series. His articles have appeared in *Prevention Magazine, Food & Wine Magazine, Eating Well, Cooking Light,* and *National Geographic Traveler Magazine*. He lives in Miami, Florida, with his wife.